"Thank you Dr. Cook for writing a book 1 complexities of endometriosis from the ҏ expert in the field, but also clearly capture‗ is like to suffer from endometriosis. Women should not have to suffer in isolation and silence. They should demand—and get—correct diagnoses and proper effective treatment, not mistreatment and unnecessary invasive procedures. This book is a most welcome source of hope for women to break open the taboos about discussing endometriosis and get the medical community to recognize their obligation to rethink how this disease is treated."

—Susan Sarandon, actress

"Endometriosis is a complex disease that requires a multidimensional management approach from knowledgeable professionals who are committed to their patients. Andrew Cook is just such a physician and surgeon whose book provides expert and comprehensive advice that will benefit many patients."

—G. David Adamson MD, FRCSC, FACOG, FACS
Director of Fertility Physicians of Northern California
Adjunct Clinical Professor at Stanford University
Clinical Associate Professor at the University of
California, San Francisco

"*Stop Endometriosis and Pelvic Pain* is the single most accurate and helpful guide available for dealing effectively with this common problem. Bravo, Dr. Cook!"

—Christiane Northrup MD
OB/GYN physician and author of the *New York Times* bestsellers: *Women's Bodies, Women's Wisdom* and *The Wisdom of Menopause*

"This book is the long-awaited blessing for the millions of women who faced limited options in dealing with endometriosis and pelvic pain. It will no doubt become the most authoritative text offering a comprehensive, integrative approach to these issues for clinician and patient alike. Dr. Cook provides the answers we have been waiting for."

—David Perlmutter MD, FACN, ABIHM
Author of *Power Up Your Brain, The Neuroscience of Enlightenment*

Stop Endometriosis
AND Pelvic Pain

Stop Endometriosis
AND Pelvic Pain

What Every Woman and Her Doctor Need to Know

Andrew S. Cook MD, FACOG

Femsana Press
LOS GATOS, CALIFORNIA

Important Note to Readers

This publication should not be used as a substitute for professional medical advice or care. The reader should consult a physician in matters relating to her health. In particular, the reader should consult with a competent professional before undertaking any form of self-treatment or acting on any of the information or advice contained in this book.

Modifying a medical regimen can be very dangerous. Any side effects should be reported promptly to the physician. A reader concerned about adverse effects of any medical evaluation or treatment should discuss with her doctor the benefits as well as the risks of receiving the medical evaluation or treatment.

The information contained in this book regarding health and and medical treatments is the result of extensive personal clinical experience with patients as well as reviews of relevant medical and scientific literature. That literature at times reflects conflicting conclusions and opinions. The author has expressed his view on many of those issues; the reader should understand that other experts might disagree. The author and publisher specifically disclaim any and all liability arising directly or indirectly from the use or application of any information contained in this book.

Publisher's Cataloging-in-Publication data

Cook, Andrew S.
    Stop endometriosis and pelvic pain : what every woman and her doctor need to know / Andrew S. Cook, MD, FACOG.
        p. cm.
        ISBN 9780984953578 (pbk)
        ISBN 9780984953509 (e-book)
        Includes bibliographical references and index.
    1. Endometriosis. 2. Endometriosis—Treatment. 3. Pelvic pain. 4. Pelvic pain—Treatment.
    5. Pelvis—Diseases—Treatment. 6. Menstruation disorders—Treatment. I. Title.

RG483.E53 C66 2012
618.1—dc23   2012935941

Printed in the United States of America
The last digit is the print number: 9 8 7 6 5 4 3 2

Book design: Hae Yuon Kim of Tobi Designs
Cover design: Alicia Buelow
Graphic illustrations: Andrew S. Cook
Primary editing: Pamela Feinsilber
Secondary editing, indexing, and project management by
    Marla Wilson of Printed Page Productions

*This book is dedicated to all the women
who have suffered with endometriosis and pelvic pain.
My hope is that this book will help you better
understand this disease and guide you in your journey
to regain your health.*

ACKNOWLEDGMENTS

This book is a result of much more than my efforts. It has been made possible only through the efforts of many people.

I would like to recognize all the members of the healthcare team that make up Vital Health Institute. VHI has been called a model for the treatment of endometriosis and pelvic pain, and for good healthcare in general. The quality of healthcare and compassion provided at Vital Health comes from more than just myself; it is truly a team effort.

I would like to thank my wonderful staff, including Linda Mavity NP, Danielle Cook MS, RD, CDE, Michelle Waterstreet, Margaret Sterner, Gabrielle Terrado RN, Neesha Tatla, Ted Sterner, Jil Britt, and Mary Notario.

Several healthcare professionals contributed information for this book. Douglas Drucker PhD, is a psychologist who specializes in helping women with chronic pain in their recovery process. Amy Day ND, is a naturopathic doctor who appreciates the multidisciplinary approach in treating endometriosis and pelvic pain. Amy Cooper PhD, is a sexologist who helps women reconnect with their sexuality. Previous employees of Vital Health Institute, Lene Joy, a nutritionist, and Mark Howard DO and functional medicine physician, both made helpful contributions.

Many endometriosis and pelvic-pain patients and even some of their spouses made generous contributions to this book. Among them I would like to thank Lillyth, Elizabeth, Gabrielle, Lisa, Kelly, Shannon, Connie, Jeff, Kari, John (Mendo), I-Li, Kathleen, Keala, Kelli, Bessy, Michele, Erika, Peggy, and Roy. Please accept my heartfelt thanks and deep gratitude for your help.

I would also like to acknowledge several mentors who were instrumental in both guiding me to the field of endometriosis and helping me hone my skills: Robert Franklin MD ("the grandfather of endometriosis"), a kind man and outstanding surgeon who inspired me to follow in his footsteps and dedicate my life to treating women with endometriosis and pelvic pain; Robert Kelly MD, the first surgeon in the United States to use laparoscopy and the CO_2 laser to treat endometriosis and who was instrumental in developing my surgical skills; David Adamson MD, one of the most honest and hardworking physicians I know, who I had the privilege to work with when starting out in practice and who has been a friend over the last 20 years. He was also influential in developing my surgical skills.

Thanks also to Joe Keon PhD, friend, mentor, and author of the critically acclaimed book *Whitewash*, for his input and the significant time he provided, including reviewing the manuscript and making insightful comments.

I would also like to thank Laura Fraser for her thoughtful contributions and Pamela Feinsilber for a very detailed editing process to help make this book as readable and clear as possible. I would also like to acknowledge Marla Wilson for her help on this project, not only in indexing the book and providing editorial comments, but also for overseeing all the details in getting this book to press. Finally, I would like to thank Alicia Buelow for creating such a beautiful cover.

CONTENTS

PART III: PUTTING IT ALL TOGETHER

FIGURES

TABLES

FOREWORD

During my 60 years of practicing medicine, I have treated over 20,000 women with endometriosis, a complex disease that can rob women of a functional life. When I first started treating endometriosis, most people, including physicians had never heard of it. The word about this disease is slowly getting out, but the current approach most medical doctors use to treat endo is lacking. There is much confusion and many misperceptions about endo, even within the medical community. As a group, physicians are currently without a clear and comprehensive mandate for diagnosis and treatment. Patients frequently don't know where to turn for the best treatment, and as a result, needlessly endure long periods of pain.

Stop Endometriosis and Pelvic Pain: What Every Woman and Her Doctor Need to Know is a book that has long needed to be written. It gathers together what is known about endometriosis and presents a practical approach to the treatment.

Dr. Cook has a deep understanding of this complex disease, gleaned from years of experience as a gynecologist who focuses on a comprehensive approach to treating complex cases of endometriosis, both surgically and non-surgically, along with his habit of listening closely to his patients. He has presented the latest medical understanding about endometriosis and provided a practical and understandable approach to treatment. Any woman who has endometriosis, or who is suspected of having the disease, should read this book. Dr. Cook's book will also be an invaluable resource for anyone who cares for these patients, including physicians.

I have come to believe that endometriosis should be a separate specialty in obstetrics and gynecology. Unfortunately, the current official guidelines for treatment of endometriosis are done by committee and, as is common in this type of situation, comes out with a very bland and non-committal approach to treating endometriosis. This is not helpful in promoting a better understanding and treatment of this disease. Because there is no official endometriosis specialty, it's important for patients to know how to identify a physician who can provide the best care for the disease. Too often, patients who seek care end up in the hands of the wrong physician, with the wrong diagnosis, and the wrong treatment. This book will help patients with endometriosis understand what to look for in a physician and how to find the best care they need.

Endometriosis is a disease that affects many systems in the body and shows up in different patients in different ways. That's why, as Dr. Cook clearly describes in his book, it is important to have a team of health care professionals. Patients may need to see bowel surgeons, gastroenterologists, endocrinologists, immunologists, and other physicians. Dr. Cook also brings psychologists and complementary healthcare providers into the mix, to help his patients manage the disease in all aspects of their lives. It's vital that patients have a physician who can coordinate that care and who understands the big picture of her health.

Dr. Cook also explains, in clear detail, why it's important to have a specialist do endometriosis surgery. During surgery, the physician has to meticulously remove all the endometriosis, a skill that requires years of training and experience. After surgery, the physician needs to evaluate the patient to see what symptoms are still present and work with other specialists to ensure that the non-surgical aspects of this disease are cleared up and health is restored.

One of Dr. Cook's biggest contributions with this book is his emphasis on listening to, and working with, his patients. He tries to form a relationship with each patient that will make her realize that he's working with her, but at the same time her participation in her health is essential. As outlined in the book, one of the first things a physician dealing with endometriosis has to do is develop a rapport with their patient, which allows him or her to adequately study, understand, and treat each patient's unique situation.

This is the moment of truth for the medical community to step up and honestly address the issues of how women with endometriosis are treated. I hope physicians as well as endometriosis sufferers read this book, spread the book, and demand better care. I am glad that Dr. Cook has brought this useful, thorough, compassionate, and much-needed book to the public.

Robert Franklin MD
Clinical Professor of OB/GYN
Baylor College of Medicine
Houston, Texas
May 2012

INTRODUCTION

The Overlooked Endo Patient

Endometriosis is a complicated, debilitating disease that is poorly understood and all too frequently misdiagnosed. Most of the patients I see have suffered from excruciating pain for years. Added to that pain is frustration, because many of the people in their lives—doctors, colleagues, even husbands or partners—dismiss their symptoms as exaggerated or "all in her head." These women put on a brave face, but they are increasingly worn down—by pain, by rounds of treatments, and even surgery that brings little relief, by a medical system in which they feel increasingly disappointed, by struggling to maintain a normal work and family life, by the despair that comes from losing hope that they will ever feel well again.

I'm writing this book, first of all, for women who have endometriosis, to explain what we know about this mysterious disease, to dispel some myths, to help you realize you're not alone, and, above all, to offer hope. More than 5.5 million women in North America[1] and 176 million women worldwide[2] suffer from endometriosis, and far too many of them receive inadequate treatment. Because so few doctors specialize in this complex disease, the average time from onset of symptoms to diagnosis ranges from 7.96 years in the United Kingdom

---

1   Endometriosis Page. U.S. Department of Health and Human Services Public Health Service National Institutes of Health Eunice Kennedy Shriver National Institute of Child Health and Human Development. http://www.nichd.nih.gov/publications/pubs/endometriosis. Updated 3/30/2010. Accessed June 12, 2011.

2   Adamson GD, Kennedy SH, Hummelshoj L. Creating solutions in endometriosis: Global collaboration through the World Endometriosis Research Foundation. J Endometriosis 2010;2:3 -6.

to 11.73 years in the United States.[3] It can take years after that to find appropriate treatment.

In fact, effective treatments *are* available that can make women with endometriosis healthy and active again. After endometriosis surgery, most of my patients have gone back to their normal lives, many living without pain. Their endo has not come back; they are in remission, and it is possible that they may be cured, never to experience endo again.

Because endometriosis is so difficult to diagnose, endometriosis is not currently a sub-specialty, and so few general OB/GYN doctors know how to treat this disease properly, it can be hard to find effective, respectful medical care. But it's essential. You have to educate yourself about this frustrating disease and find the support to cope with it. You need a physician who won't make you think you're crazy for reporting severe pain symptoms for which he or she can't find a cause or cure. Your doctor should listen to you, treat you with respect, give you a thorough exam, clearly explain your medical and surgical options, and provide you with adequate pain relief. In addition, your physician should offer suggestions for improving your overall health and well-being through nutrition, exercise, and perhaps complementary therapies. Most important, your doctor should be an expert in the surgical techniques that remove endometriosis—the only way to rid yourself of this disease.

I'm also writing this book for the people who love, support, or work with a woman who has endometriosis. It's not easy when someone you are close to is in constant, sometimes debilitating, pain. It can make you feel helpless, frustrated, angry, and sad. I hope this book will help you understand more about the disease, so that you can better support that woman in your life.

I dedicate this book to the thousands of women with endometriosis who have been misdiagnosed, ignored, treated as hypochondriacs or complainers, sent to psychiatrists instead of to surgeons, and otherwise

---

3   Hadfield R, Mardon H, Barlow D, Kennedy S. Delay in the diagnosis of endometriosis: a survey of women from the USA and the UK. *Human Reproduction*. 1996;11(4):878-880.

dismissed. As a man, I can't imagine the pain you've endured, just as I can't imagine the pain of childbirth. But as a physician who has seen women's pelvic regions peppered with the blisters, scars, and cysts caused by endometriosis, I know that pain is all too terribly real. I also know that it can be treated. You may have to be proactive to find appropriate care; you may even have to travel to get the best treatment possible. But good care is out there, as well as good information and support.

With proper treatment, the vast majority of women with endometriosis and pelvic pain will have a significant reduction or elimination of their pain. At this time most women, unfortunately, are not being provided with this level of care. It is my belief that the changes needed to provide better care for all endometriosis patients will be a grass roots effort resulting from women refusing to tolerate the current mediocre treatment for endometriosis. Women empowered with knowledge, the Internet, and social media can be the driving force to demand and achieve the required changes to improve the standard of care provided by physicians to patients with endometriosis and pelvic pain. With all the incredible advances in medical technology over the past few years, surely it's time for a more modern understanding of endometriosis and more compassionate and respectful treatment.

Treatment of endometriosis and pelvic pain can be challenging and complex. The time is overdue for treatment of endometriosis to be recognized as a sub-specialty with all of the associated specialized expertise and quality-of-care accountability afforded by an official medical sub-speciality. Contrary to current practices, general OB/GYNs without specialized expertise should not be expected to provide the care needed by endometriosis patients. It is not fair to the general OB/GYN doctor, and it certainly is not fair to the endometriosis patient.

PART I

The Reality
OF Endometriosis
and Pelvic Pain

CHAPTER ONE

What It Really Means to Have Endometriosis

From a medical point of view, endometriosis is defined as a disease whereby the inside lining of the uterus, the endometrium, somehow implants and grows outside the uterus. Endometriosis lesions, which are like blisters, can be found anywhere in the pelvic cavity, including in all the reproductive organs, the bladder, bowel, intestines, colon, appendix, and rectum. Endometriosis can also cause scar tissue (adhesions), which can make internal tissues sticky and sometimes even cause internal organs to fuse together. The hallmark of endometriosis is severe pain. It can also cause infertility.

So much for the medical definition of endometriosis. In my experience treating women with pelvic pain—more than 25 years of residency, private practice, and fellowship—the medical definition doesn't even come close to describing what it's like to experience this disease.

Having endometriosis is like having tens or hundreds of excruciatingly painful blisters or bee stings covering the inside of your pelvis. We all know how painful a small blister on the foot can be, and how sore the surrounding tissue is. When you're hiking with a blister on your heel, every step can cause a sharp pain. A blister on your hand from a cooking burn can bother you for weeks, every time you accidentally touch it. Now imagine those blisters multiplied and multiplied, spread throughout your internal organs; picture the entire pelvic area red, raw, and sore. When the blisters ooze, they can spread to form other blisters, like poison oak does. Any jostling or movement aggravates the pain.

If you can imagine those blisters, perhaps you can better understand how women with endometriosis (endo for short) can feel intense, horrific pain that few of us, we hope, will ever have to experience. Some women describe it as worse than labor pains: knifelike stabs in the pelvis, aching, stinging, and burning. The pain isn't limited to the uterine area; it can be side pain, ovarian pain, hip pain, thigh pain, and fairly severe lower-back pain. It can be grinding pain, like that experienced by advanced cancer patients. In addition, women can experience nausea, pain with intercourse or bowel movements, flulike symptoms, and general fatigue. Endometriosis can truly be torture.

I think the closest way a man can relate is to imagine getting hit in the testicles on a regular basis. If men were describing that kind of pain to their physicians, I'm guessing they'd be taken a lot more seriously than are many women who complain of the pain from endo.

And, of course, being with someone who's unable to live a normal life is hard on her partner as well. Let John Blondin, the husband of a woman with endo, who created a group for men in his situation, Mendo,[4] describe the challenges endometriosis can bring to a relationship:

> "Endo means loss—loss of many of the things I had hoped for with this relationship. It means the loss of not just sex but the physical contact between a man and a woman. It means that my wife no longer feels she can touch me in any way. Not because she does not want to, but because, as she says, 'It is hard to feel good when I hurt so bad.' The more she hurts, the deeper she withdraws within to protect herself. She feels she can no longer extend herself in any way that could remotely be considered sexual, because 'I don't want to start anything that I can't finish; it's not fair to you.'

> "It means that I come home from work and do not know what I will find. Will she be lying in bed in a fetal position, face wet from the tears of frustration and pain? Will I find her sitting on the couch, trying to show a cheerful façade,

---

4   Blondin J. Communications: one way to understand endometriosis. http://endometriosis. org/resources/articles/communications-to-understand-endometriosis. Accessed June 12, 2011.

a facsimile of what she used to be? Will I find her dressed, dinner ready, the house clean, but she collapses in my arms when I hug her because she is so worn out from the effort? Bursting into tears because she cannot do the things she used to and she knows that I am tired but will do them for her?

"Endo means that I have to be second in this, because I am healthy. It means that I have to do the things that need to be done so that she will not feel that she has to. Endo means that I cannot do anything to make the pain go away. It means that I sit and hold her, stroke her hair, and try my best to make her feel better, knowing that I am doing virtually nothing that makes a difference in the way she feels, though I am probably making her feel more secure. It means I have to learn to keep to myself the anger, frustration, and tears, because she has enough to deal with. It means I have to be strong, someone she can lean on, even though I am dying inside.

"Endo means that we cannot plan to do anything—outings, walks, anything. It means that doing something spur of the moment is a rare and wonderful thing. Endo means problems having children: because she cannot conceive and because, most of the time, we cannot even make love. It means the possibility that we may never have children hangs over us like an ominous cloud. Endometriosis means that the lives we had planned and wished for now are just that: wishes."

How Does Endometriosis Start?

Most women with endo begin to have pain in their teenage years, sometimes even starting in elementary school as a "tween." While similar in timing, this pain is completely different from mild menstrual cramps many women without endometriosis experience. It is not uncommon for these girls to miss a couple of days of school each month from cyclic pain that can be worse than the level of pain experienced after major surgery.

This, of course, is the time to begin to suspect and treat endometriosis. But because there's a general lack of awareness of the disease, many of these girls don't get a correct diagnosis or any support. Many families, knowing nothing about endometriosis, believe the girls are suffering menstrual cramps that are in the realm of normal, and are perhaps exaggerating the pain. In some families, there's a tendency not to discuss "private parts" and "women's problems," and often, girls who feel embarrassed about their newly changing bodies haven't learned how to stand up for themselves and say that something really hurts.

The girls may also be ignored because there's a natural tendency to think girls that age can be overdramatic or are just avoiding school. In what may be the first episode in a decades-long pattern of frustration, the girl's symptoms are invalidated. Her family and physician may even suggest that psychological issues are driving the severity of her pain. When the girl hears the message that the pain isn't serious or real, what she really is learning is to distrust her senses, her body—and herself. Worse, it may affect her self-esteem, as she comes to believe that others don't think her devastating pain is worth their trouble.

But believe me, that girl's pain is real, and it's nothing like the periodic cramping most teenage girls experience occasionally.

Here's how a few of my patients—the real experts—describe their early experience with pelvic pain:

> "At the age of 11, I started my period, and the pain was tough. 'It's just cramps,' my mom would say. I grew up thinking that being a woman meant monthly pain, that suffering is part of being female. The doctor repeated my mother's decree: it's just female issues, so deal with it." —I-Li

> "At age 15 the pain I lived with every month started to get worse. My grandmother had called this pain normal—a discomfort that women were sentenced to by Eve in the Garden of Eden. My family practitioner had no idea what

was causing my discomfort. I couldn't walk very far, and for a young body, there was no excuse for that. The pain was ruining my life." —Lillyth

"I was the daughter who repeatedly collapsed from pain. Instead of nurturing me, my mother got tough. Instead of taking me to the doctor, she taught me to bear the circumstances. In college, I was in pain much of the time—deep pelvic pain that would cause me to vomit—but I did not see a doctor until later, because I was taught that it was all in my head." —Lisa

How Does the Disease Progress?

Unlike with mild menstrual cramps, the pain with endometriosis increases. With my patients, a typical history is starting her period at 11 or 12; for a couple of years the pain isn't too bad; her periods start getting worse, eventually causing her to miss a day of school, a couple of days; then the pain is constant. Both the severity and duration of the pain typically progress until she has more nonfunctioning days than normal days. The pain becomes so severe and unpredictable that on many days she can't do anything but stay in bed. There can be so many of those days that she can't maintain a normal schedule.

For some women with endo, the pain is severe for just a couple of days during their period, but in the worst cases, they never feel real relief. The pain affects their ability to function in a normal manner—professionally, personally, and in relationships. Then things begin to snowball: they miss more and more work because of their pain; they may lose their jobs and thus their health insurance. They feel so crummy they can't work out; they're so nauseated they eat only carbohydrates in an effort not to feel sick; they start to gain weight; they feel horrible all the time; and a once lively woman is now doing her best to simply exist. It's a very sad picture.

Women with endo may get to the point where they can no longer rely on their bodies. They can't make a simple date for tennis next Thursday or a dinner party on Friday, because they don't know whether they'll be in bed doubled up in pain. They're tired of making excuses to their friends about such a private problem. It becomes increasingly difficult to make any plans when it's likely they won't be able to follow through.

Endometriosis can take away many, even most, aspects of a normal life. Mothers can't reliably meet the needs of their children. Women with jobs outside the home can't get to work and function at their highest capacity. Wives push through the pain to be intimate with their husbands, but eventually the pain becomes too intense. Being the loving, compassionate woman, mother, and partner that she truly is becomes more and more difficult. Feeling like a vibrant and desirable being is often a dim memory. The pain takes over her life, and the stress on family relationships is common and real.

Added to the physical pain is the guilt these women carry for not being able to fulfill the many roles in their lives and the frustration they feel when no one believes them or is able to help them. A woman who has endo often lacks the energy to pursue her passions, goals, dreams, and commitments. It's hard for her to imagine being the creative person she once was, filled with ideas and energy. She can end up feeling she's failing to live at all.

Even in this state, most women continue to fight the disease, refusing to let it completely take over their lives. That fight often entails many rounds of medical visits and unsuccessful treatments; that alone can wear a woman down. Yet you can meet a woman who has endo and have no idea of the devastating illness she's dealing with. Most of the time, these women get up, put on a brave face, and try to live normal lives. Even when pain relievers don't touch their pain, they have no choice but to carry on the best they can.

The Invisible Disease

One of the problems with endometriosis is that it is a silent and invisible disease. If you have rheumatoid arthritis, people around you see your gnarled hands and think, "No wonder they hurt." If you're in a cast or covered in bandages, people understand the grimace on your face. But with endo, the cause of the pain is hidden, so it is all too easy for people to blame the woman, not the disease—and for the woman to blame herself, against all reason, for not getting better. With this disease, the woman is effectively held prisoner and tortured by her own body in broad daylight, often with no one who fully understands her situation or who can effectively help her.

Because endo is invisible, and because few physicians are specialists in the disease, it is frequently overlooked or misdiagnosed. The typical woman who ends up in my office has been through many physicians, and usually several types of treatments and surgeries, and has not found real relief from her pain. Often, she's jaded about the medical community: she doesn't feel she's been listened to; her experiences have been dismissed; she's frustrated that a system she believed would heal her hasn't worked. She's at the end of her considerable patience.

By the time they get to me, the women often have symptoms like those of Post-Traumatic Stress Disorder, on top of the endometriosis. They've been through so much unnecessary pain, yet they're afraid to talk straight about their problems because people have disbelieved them so often. They're fatigued, fed up, scared, despairing, and operating as mere shadows of themselves.

If you want the real definition of endometriosis, you can't find it in a medical dictionary. You have to listen to the patients and believe what they're saying—and too few people have taken the time to do that.

Why Is It So Hard to Find Good Care for Pelvic Pain and Endometriosis?

As a patient, you expect that when you go to a doctor, the person in the white coat will have a complete understanding of your medical condition and the best way to treat it. After all, doctors have gone through more years of schooling than people in most any other profession; they should be experts in their field. Unfortunately, this is all too often not the case with endometriosis and pelvic pain. But why?

When it comes to treating endometriosis, the entire system seems to be broken. In a way, we are all victims of this broken system, including the general OB/GYN doctors, the medical societies that make questionable treatment recommendations,[5] even the insurance companies that in the long run pay much more to treat this disease than is necessary.

An OB/GYN physician is expected to take care of a wide variety of female health-related issues. They are considered primary-care physicians (rather than specialists), as are those who work in the areas of family practice, internal medicine, and pediatrics. Specialists are doctors whom you visit for a specific, complex problem, such as cardiologists for heart disease. There are four OB/GYN subspecialties: high-risk pregnancy, gynecological cancer, infertility, and bladder or prolapse problems. There is no endometriosis or pelvic-pain specialty.

Yet the complexity of this disease—endometriosis and pelvic pain—fully warrants a subspecialty. The information and skills needed to treat heart disease well is the reason for the specialty in cardiology. Imagine if there were no cardiologists, and internal-medicine doctors had to treat heart disease along with the colds and other illnesses they normally deal with. It's easy to see that the quality of care for heart patients would suffer.

If you went to an internal-medicine doctor with a heart problem, he or she would more likely refer you to a cardiology specialist than to another internal-medicine physician (and thus a competitor), even if that physician had the same knowledge base and skill set as a cardiologist. Similarly, a general OB/GYN is reluctant to refer a patient to another OB/GYN, even when some OB/GYNs have much more experience in treating endometriosis.

I've found that many OB/GYN doctors do not believe effective treatments are available for endometriosis or that endometriosis specialists have anything significant to offer. They couldn't be more wrong. Physicians who have devoted their lives to patients with endo and pelvic pain can provide better and more effective treatment than most general OB/GYNs. Physicians who have specialized in advanced operative laparoscopy for the treatment of endometriosis and pelvic pain

---

5   Practice bulletin no. 114: Management of endometriosis. *Obstetrics and Gynecology*. 2010;116(1):223-236.

provide a whole different form of surgical treatment. The specialists who offer a multidisciplinary approach provide even more comprehensive treatment.

Consider the results of a survey commissioned by the United Kingdom's Endometriosis All-Party Parliamentary Group and presented at the Ninth World Congress on Endometriosis in 2005. The Pain and Quality of Life Survey looked at 7,025 women from 52 countries. The data showed that surgery by OB/GYNs who are not specialists in endometriosis was, in general, not very effective.[6] Of the 5,478 women who had had surgery from nonspecialist OB/GYNs, 4 percent felt the surgery was very effective; 4 percent, moderately effective; 22 percent, slightly effective—a total of 30 percent who felt at least some improvement. That left fully 70 percent of the patients saying their surgeries were ineffective or whose outcomes were worse than before the surgery.

Other data from the Ninth World Congress on Endometriosis revealed that hormonal treatment, such as birth control pills and medications containing GnRH agonists, such as Lupron, was at least slightly effective in 37 percent of the 5,669 women treated with these medications. This means that hormonal therapy for endometriosis is more effective than the surgical treatment offered by general OB/GYNs. That probably accounts for the perception among many OB/GYNs that medical treatment is as effective as surgery. It may also explain why the American College of Obstetrics and Gynecology, in the Practice Bulletin on the management of endometriosis (July 2010) equally supports GnRH agonists and surgery for treatment of endo.

An alternative not mentioned in the Practice Bulletin is referring the patient to a surgeon who specializes in the treatment of endometriosis. Studies presented at the Ninth World Congress on Endometriosis showed that women who were treated by surgeons who specialize in endometriosis had up to 80 percent improvement in pain levels, quality of life, and sexual activity.[7]

---

6   Pain and Quality of Life Survey, commissioned by the UK Endometriosis All-Party Parliamentary Group and presented at the Ninth World Congress on Endometriosis, Maastricht, The Netherlands, 2005.

7   Abbott J, Hawe J, Hunter D, Holmes M, Finn P, Garry R. Laparoscopic excision of endometriosis: a randomized, placebo-controlled trial. *Fertility Sterility*. 2004;82(4):878-884.

These findings are similar to ours at the Vital Health Institute. We have just completed a rigorous process of data entry and statistical analysis of our outcomes from over 600 endometriosis surgeries, which I have performed over the last 10 years. We send out questionnaires to our patients every 3 months the first year after surgery and then every subsequent year. The length of follow-up currently varies from 3 months to 9 years.

An initial review of the data shows that, on average, patients had 3.4 surgeries before coming to VHI and receiving surgery from me. Afterward, when asked what percent better they are then prior to surgery, on average they report a 75 percent improvement with 57 percent of patients experiencing between 90 and 100 percent improvement. Broken down into quartiles, 7 percent of patients experience 0 to 25 percent improvement, 9 percent of patients 25 to 50 percent improvement, 17 percent of patients 50 to 75 percent improvement, and 67 percent of patients 75 to 100 percent improvement. The reoperation rate—the number of patients undergoing more than one surgery—is 16 percent and the recurrence rate—how often endo is found at a repeat surgery—is substantially lower than the reoperation rate.

Treatment of endometriosis usually requires more than just surgery, but surgery performed correctly is an integral part of a successful and effective endometriosis treatment program.

This is not a hopeless disease that cannot be treated, but too often it is a disease with a hopeless outcome resulting from poor treatment. I have seen so many women suffering needlessly. The system needs to change. How do we do this?

To start with, we simply need to open our minds and educate ourselves. Then we need to demand more effective treatment. Early referral to a pelvic-pain and endometriosis specialist, particularly when treatment by a general OB/GYN has not been effective, should, in my opinion, be the standard of care.

As a patient suffering from endometriosis and pelvic pain, you need to stand up for yourself. Do not stop until you get the treatment you need and deserve.

CHAPTER TWO

The Medical Mystery of Endometriosis

What Causes Endometriosis?

Endometriosis is the presence of endometrial tissue outside the uterus, the organ in which a baby grows during pregnancy. Physicians and researchers don't know why this occurs in some women, but we do have some theories. Let me give you some medical background on this disease.

The most widely held theory as to what causes endo is called retrograde menstruation. Menstrual tissue, which normally flows out the vagina, sometimes flows backwards through the fallopian tubes and deposits on the pelvic organs, where it can grow, causing painful blisters and scars. Endo may also travel by other means, through blood vessels or the lymph system—which is how, very rarely, endo ends up in distant parts of the body, such as the lungs or spinal column. Endometrial tissue can also spread through surgery, particularly following a Cesarean section. The "coelomic metaplasia theory" suggests that it's not so much a matter of the endometrial tissue traveling from the uterus but of residual embryonic tissue in the pelvis somehow changing into endometrial tissue once a woman starts menstruating and making estrogen.

There is probably some truth to all the theories, but let's focus on retrograde menstruation, since this is the most common and widely accepted one. Researchers have found that about 90 percent of all women have retrograde flow. Yet only a relatively small percentage develop endometriosis. Why? Many questions about retrograde menstruation remain unanswered, and this is the biggest one.

Normally, the endometrium—a thin layer of glands lining the uterus, which, during pregnancy, provides nutritional support to the fetus prior to the development of the placenta—grows during the first half of the menstrual cycle. It is fed by estrogen, a female hormone. After ovulation occurs (about two weeks after the first day of bleeding), the other female hormone, progesterone, kicks in, to help stabilize and mature the endometrial lining. If a woman is not pregnant, both estrogen and progesterone levels drop at the end of her menstrual cycle, the endometrial lining sloughs off, and her period—the menses flowing out of the body through the vagina—starts the next day. When a woman has mild cramping during her period, the uterus is producing painful prostaglandins and contracting in reaction to clots of blood in the uterus. This is completely unrelated to the cramping caused by endo.

Why Are Some Women More Susceptible Than Others?

Researchers don't have a solid idea about why some women get endometriosis and others don't. A lot of things probably come into play, including a woman's immune system and the amount of tissue that her body has to get rid of each month. A few possible contributing factors follow.

Genetics

Studies show that a woman who has a first-degree relative (mother or sister) who has endometriosis is more likely to develop the disease herself. One study shows that the risk of endometriosis appears to follow the mother's side of the family, and that women with a first-degree relative with endo are more likely to have severe disease than someone without a family history.[8]

---

8   Lamb K, Hoffman RG, Nichols TR. Family trait analysis: a case-control study of 43 women with endometriosis and their best friends. *American Journal of Obstetrics and Gynecology*. 1986;154(3):596-601.

Other research studies have tried to define the genes responsible for endometriosis, by looking at DNA mapping or associated genes. It seems there are significant alterations in gene expression.[9] Once the particular genes are discovered, it likely will be easier to come up with a noninvasive diagnostic test for the disease, and perhaps improved treatment as well.[10]

The fact that endometriosis has a genetic component doesn't explain what causes the disease, just that it runs in families. But the research means that if your sister or mother has had endometriosis and you have pelvic pain, you want to make sure you let your physician know about your family history, so that you get appropriate treatment. Someday—soon, we hope—genetic research will offer us easier diagnostic and treatment tools for this difficult disease.

Epigenetics and Epigenomics
Each of us has a unique genetic makeup. How the environment interacts with our genetic makeup plays a significant role in our health and our ability to fight disease. Not all of our genes are activated; many genes are turned off and not functioning. The interaction with our environment is a big part of what determines which genes are turned on. Epigenetics focuses on processes that control a single gene being turned on or off while epigenomics refers to the analysis of all epigenetic changes of many genes in a cell or the entire person. This subject is the focus of an emerging area of medicine known as epigenomic medicine. The National Institutes of Health (NIH) announced in 2008 that it would be investing more than $190 million over the next five years to accelerate the field of epigenomics.[11]

At one time, we might have thought that since endometriosis has a genetic component, it cannot be prevented or the risk reduced of it

---

9   Hansen KA, Eyster KM. Genetics and genomics of endometriosis. *Clinical Obstetrics & Gynecology*. 2010;53(2):403-412.

10   For more information on the genetics of endometriosis, or to participate in the Genetic Endometriosis Research Study, contact Juneau Biosciences. http://www.endtoendo.com

11   Press Release, *NIH Announces New Initiative in Epigenomics*. U.S. Department of Health and Services, NIH News, National Institutes of Health. http://www.nih.gov/news/health/jan2008/od-22.htm. Updated January 22, 2008. Accessed June 12, 2011.

being passed down to daughters of patients with endometriosis. But the new field of epigenomics suggests that things in your environment, including the foods you eat, may activate dormant genes or possibly even make you more susceptible to developing endometriosis. A recent scientific study was one of the first to look at epigenetic differences in gene regulation between patients with and without endometriosis. The findings of this study "support the notion that endometriosis may be an epigenetic disease."[12] Scientists feel we will gain major insight into the cause of endometriosis, as this area of research is being extensively studied over the next 2 to 5 years.[13] Essentially, how you live might affect your susceptibility to the disease. Cutting-edge science suggests that nutrition and exercise can affect the disease-activating genes. I am not saying that junk food causes endo. But if you live a healthier life, you may be able to modify your epigenomic expression or gene activity.

Even more exciting, it's possible that this improvement in epigenomics may actually be passed on to your children, which means they might become less susceptible to endo as well. It's too early to say definitively—all this is very new science and little understood—but the notion that your lifestyle could affect your genes is one more argument for living in a way that keeps you as healthy as possible.

Environmental Exposure

This is an area in which we need a great deal of research, but it could offer promising clues about this disease. Studies in rhesus monkeys have shown that environmental pollutants can increase the risk of endometriosis, just as they have been shown to increase the risk of certain cancers. In one 1992 study, researchers found that 79 percent of monkeys that were exposed to an environmental pollutant called dioxin developed endometriosis, while those who were not exposed

---

12 van Kaam Kj, Delvoux B, Romano A, D'Hooghe T, Dunselman GA, Groothuis PG. Deoxyribonucleic acid methyltransferases and methyl-CpG-binding domain proteins in human endometrium and endometriosis. *Fertility and Sterility*. 2011;Feb 12 (Epub ahead of print).

13 Giudice LC. Hot topics in basic research in endometriosis. *World Endometriosis Society e-Journal*. 2011;13(2):3-5.

to dioxin had very little or no disease. There was a direct correlation: the more dioxin exposure in the individual monkey, the greater the endometriosis.[14]

Dairy is the second largest contributor of dioxin in our diet.[15] Researchers speculate that women who don't have endometriosis have immune cells in the peritoneal cavity that destroy endometrial cells or discourage their growth. The presence of dioxins and other chemicals may change how this immune response functions, which can result in the unregulated growth of endometrial cells. Other research has shown that dioxins and other pollutants can disrupt how hormones work, which could also contribute to endometriosis.

We do not completely understand the scientific relationship between lifestyle, environment, and endometriosis. Clearly, the interaction of environmental toxins, hormonal disruption, and endometriosis is one that needs more research. But given that environmental pollutants may increase your risk of endo, the question comes down to this: how can you reduce exposure to the environmental pollutants that may contribute to the disease?

Here are a few suggestions, which apply to preventing cancer, too:[16]

- Eat organic as often as possible, since foods that have been grown without toxic chemicals are healthier by far.

- Avoid dairy products.

- Avoid contaminated fish; dioxins are concentrated in the dark stripe of the fish.

- Filter your water to make sure that the PCBs, lead, mercury, and chlorine are removed.

- Switch to chlorine-free paper products, including tampons and sanitary napkins, if possible.

---

14 Rier SE, Martin DC, Bowman RE, Dmowski WP, Becker JL. Endometriosis in rhesus monkeys (Macaca mulatta) following chronic exposure to 2,3,7,8-tetrachlorodibenzo-p-dioxin. *Fundamental and Applied Toxicology*. 1993;21(4):433-441.

15 Keon J. *Whitewash, The Disturbing Truth About Cow's Milk and Your Health*. New Society Publishers; 2010:101-103.

16 Ballweg ML. Avoiding Dioxins and PCBs—What You Can Do, In: *The Endometriosis Sourcebook*. Chicago, IL: Contemporary Books, Inc.; 1995:393-394.

- Take off your shoes when you come into the house to avoid tracking in toxins from the outdoors.

- Keep the air in your home clean by opening windows and regularly cleaning vents and air ducts; you can also use an air purifier.

- Substitute cloth products for bleached paper products. Use cloth towels instead of paper and unbleached coffee filters.

- Use green household cleaners, or natural ones such as vinegar and baking soda.

- Get filters for your shower and your kitchen drinking water.

- Remove the plastic wrap from your dry cleaning before you get inside the house; it traps chemicals inside. Air out your dry cleaning before bringing it into the house.

Estrogen Metabolism

From an epigenetic standpoint, dioxins seem to turn on genes that promote inflammation and allergic reactions. They may also change the way your body metabolizes estrogen—the way it gets rid of it—creating more "reactive" or harmful estrogen metabolites. Endometriosis is fed by estrogen. It may be that it's not too much estrogen causing the disease, but too much of what we can think of as "bad" estrogen, the way you might think of "bad" cholesterol.[17]

How do you get bad estrogen?

When something in the body needs to be eliminated, it doesn't just disappear; it goes through a process of detoxification, or breaking down. When estrogen goes through the liver, three different enzymes break it down via the 2-, 4-, and 16-hydroxylation pathways. Researchers have suggested that if the estrogen is broken down into 16-hydroxylation or 4-hydroxylation (the latter is the worst), it becomes an

---

17   Lord R, Burdette C. Measuring Urinary Estrogen Metabolites for Cancer Risk Assessment. Metametrix Clinical Laboratory Department of Science and Education, 2006.

unstable molecule—a little like a free radical.[18] It can go around and grab other molecules, wreaking havoc on normal cell functioning. (The hormone Premarin, which the Women's Health Initiative study found to cause an increase in breast cancer, has been shown to preferentially break down through the 4-hydroxylation pathway.[19])

Naturally, we want to learn how to help the liver break estrogen down by one of the better pathways, and there's some evidence that good nutrition and food supplements may help. For example, cruciferous vegetables, such as broccoli, seem to help with good estrogen metabolism.

Immune Response

Immune disorders or defects may be another reason that some women develop endometriosis while others don't. As the studies on monkeys suggest, some dysfunction in the immune system comes into play with endometriosis. One theory is that if most women have some form of retrograde menstruation, with endometrial tissue in the pelvis, those with endo must have some sort of an autoimmune reaction to that tissue. Many women with endometriosis also suffer from other forms of autoimmune disease, such as chronic-fatigue syndrome, lupus, thyroid disease, and candida (yeast infections). Women with endo (and their families) also tend to have higher rates of allergies, food intolerances, asthma, eczema, and environmental sensitivities.[20]

Inflammation is the immune system's response to infection, injury, or irritation. Inflammation is characterized by an influx of white blood cells, gathering like an army to fight off whatever is irritating the body. Chronic inflammation, when the immune system is always activated, can lead to chronic disease. Endometriosis is a chronic disease characterized by inflammation, so anything you can do to decrease the

---

18 Prokai-Tatrai K, Prokai L. Impact of metabolism on the safety of estrogen therapy. *Annals of the New York Academy of Sciences*. 2005;1052:243-257.

19 Spink DC, Zhang F, Hussain MM, Katz BH, Liu X, Hilker DR, Bolton JL. Metabolism of equilenin in MCF-7 and MDA-MB-231 human breast cancer cells. *Chemical Research in Toxicology*. 2001;14(5):572-581.

20 Lamb K, Nichols TR. Endometriosis: a comparison of associated disease histories. American Journal of Preventive Medicine. 1986;2(6):324-329.

inflammation (for example, cut sugar, alcohol, and other inflammatory foods from your diet; we'll get to that later in the book) will help you.

If endometriosis is a disruption of the immune system, that may sound like bad news, but actually, it's an avenue of research that could lead to some hopeful discoveries. If the immune system turns out to play a strong role in endo, that information could lead to new diagnostic tools and treatment. New research could also lead to complementary treatments that might treat endo as a sort of allergic response, before it gets to the point of needing surgery. That's all in the future, but the more physicians and researchers listen to women who say they have other immune problems, the more we are going to be able to treat this disease on all fronts.

> "Along with endo, my lifelong asthma was just the tip of the iceberg. I also had undiagnosed food allergies." —Lillyth

> "I was having rashes, and the disease seemed to be affecting my immune system." —I-Li

> "Endometriosis flip-flopped a lot of things in my system. I was having immune-system problems and allergies to wheat, and it helped a lot to finally change my diet." —Kathleen

How Do I Know if I Have Endometriosis?

Endometriosis is difficult to diagnose because there's no quick test you can run, send to the lab, and wait for the results to come back positive or negative. That would make my job—and the lives of my patients— infinitely easier! This is one of the reasons endo is so frequently missed or misdiagnosed. As a specialist, I can get a good idea as to whether a patient has endo or not by listening to her describe her symptoms and performing a manual exam and a sonogram to understand the extent of her pain and disease. If you're familiar with the symptoms of endometriosis, they are fairly clear. While there are many symptoms, and some may indicate other conditions, the following symptoms usually tell me a patient has endo:

- Increasingly painful periods
- Deep pain with sexual intercourse; a patient might describe it by saying, "He's hitting something sore inside me."
- Cyclic pain that gets to the point of interfering with what you normally do in life
- Painful bowel movements

Other symptoms can include rectal pain or bleeding, blood in the urine, severe pain during periods and ovulation, back or leg pain during menstruation, sharp pain during orgasm, fatigue, infertility, cycles of constipation and diarrhea, nausea and vomiting. Endo symptoms are often worst before and during menstruation, but some women experience pain throughout their cycles.

Someday, it may be possible to diagnose endometriosis with a non-invasive immunologic test instead of laparoscopy, which is currently the only sure diagnostic method available. Right now, the physician can never make a true diagnosis until he or she looks into the pelvis through a laparoscope, which is a tube with a light in it that magnifies the area being looked at. (More on diagnosis in chapter five.)

Laparoscopy is a minor surgical procedure done under general anesthesia. The physician makes a tiny incision in the abdomen and inserts the laparoscope, distending the abdomen with carbon dioxide gas to make it easier to see inside. By moving the laparoscope around, he or she can see the endometrial implants. Normally a physician doesn't do this unless he or she strongly suspects endometriosis; once that diagnosis is confirmed, the physician usually uses the laparoscope to treat the endo as well.

Most physicians do not perform a laparotomy, opening the patient up with a "bikini cut" in the abdomen, which is how endometriosis surgery used to be done. The laparoscope offers many advantages: with its eight-fold magnification, the physician can see the diseased area more clearly; it's much easier to get into difficult areas; and recovery time is faster.

Misdiagnosis, Stigma, and Blame

In a survey by the Endometriosis Association that included 3680 of its US members with surgically diagnosed endometriosis, results showed a delay in diagnosis of almost 10 years.[21] That's 10 years of pain the women didn't need to endure. This includes the patient's delay in seeking help from a physician, for an average 4.67 years, and the physician's delay in diagnosing endometriosis, for an average 4.61 years.

A study, presented by Lone Hummelshøj at the Ninth World Congress on Endometriosis, confirmed the long delay. On average, among the 7,025 patients in this study, the diagnosis was not made until eight years after the patient first sought help from a doctor. Patients waited an average of 3 years before seeking help—for an average total of 11 years from the beginning of symptoms to diagnosis. Nearly half the patients surveyed had seen at least five different physicians before a diagnosis was made.[22]

Why does it take so long to diagnose endo? For one thing, patients often aren't taken seriously. This is in spite of the fact that so many patients I've seen are incredibly accomplished, smart professionals: CEOs, physicians, PhDs, lawyers, architects, computer scientists, graduate students, and teachers, to name a few professions. I'm amazed that so many physicians can tell such capable women that they're making up their pain, or that it's somehow psychosomatic.

The notion that pain is all in women's heads is a throwback to an age when "women's troubles" were minimized or considered invalid. Endometriosis was described early in the 1920s as "chronic abdomen," and its symptoms were remarkably like the ones we see today:

---

21 Sinaii N, Cleary SD, Ballweg ML, Nieman LK, Stratton P. High rates of autoimmune and endocrine disorders, fibromyalgia, chronic fatigue syndrome and atopic diseases among women with endometriosis: a survey analysis. *Human Reproduction.* 2002;17(10):2715-2724.

22 Pain and Quality of Life Survey, commissioned by the UK Endometriosis All-Party Parliamentary Group and presented at the Ninth World Congress on Endometriosis, Maastricht, The Netherlands, 2005.

a "raw feeling inside," a "dragging," an "indescribable sensation in the stomach," along with exhaustion and weakness. Sadly, those physicians found it tiring and frustrating to deal with patients in pain whose treatment was not easy. One particularly unkind physician of that era called the "abdominal woman" a "veritable vampire, sucking the vitality of all who come near her," and wrote, "Half an hour with her reduces her doctor to the consistence of 'a piece of chewed string,' and is more exhausting to him than all the rest of his daily visits put together, for she is always discovering fresh symptoms, will not admit any improvement in her condition, and has an objection to everything that is proposed."[23]

I wish I could say that after nearly half a century, physicians' attitudes have changed. But there are plenty of doctors who, perplexed by a patient's symptoms and uneasy about their ability to treat her, still tend to ascribe blame to the patient, not the disease. These doctors are under time pressures, and they know a patient with chronic pelvic pain is going to take a lot of their time. But there's no excuse for so many women seeing so many doctors without getting relief.

One problem with diagnosing endo is that several other maladies have some of the same symptoms. Emergency room doctors often diagnose endo as pelvic inflammatory disease (PID), which is caused by a sexually transmitted disease. Food allergies or food sensitivities can cause pains that are like the pain of endo, as can various cysts and infections. A varicose vein of your ovary can be extremely painful. Interstitial cystitis—a chronic inflammation of the bladder wall, also called painful-bladder syndrome—is sometimes diagnosed; to make matters more confusing, often both conditions might be present. Many women are misdiagnosed with irritable bowel syndrome, the catchall name for various bowel problems. Since endo can affect so many organs—the ovaries, uterus, bladder, bowel, intestines—it's not surprising that it's so often misdiagnosed.

The fact is, most physicians, even gynecologists, don't get a lot of experience during their training with this very difficult disease. Even

---

23   Hutchison R, 'The Abdominal Woman': An address on the chronic abdomen. *The British Medical Journal.* 1923;1:667-669.

physicians who *are* familiar with endometriosis often lack surgical experience. It takes a great deal of training and experience to recognize some appearances of endometriosis. The rate of negative laparoscopy—that is, of normal findings in patients with pelvic pain—has been reported to range from 21 percent to 66 percent.[24, 25, 26, 27] That's the percentage of time the doctor examines a patient with symptoms of endometriosis and does not see the endo or another anatomic cause of the pain. (In my practice, we've had negative findings less than 2 percent of the time.) This high false-negative rate may be because the doctor is looking for something obvious—like when you walk into a room and see pictures on the wall. But finding endo is more like looking for a quarter in the bed sheets when you haven't made the bed yet. Unless you pull the sheets straight and look systematically, it's easy to overlook the quarter.

Inside the pelvis, it's a lot like those rumpled sheets. When a patient is lying down, the pelvis is like a bowl; the bowel (the intestines) fills the bowl, the uterus tilts inward, and the ovaries hang down. People who do a lot of laparoscopy in the pelvis know to put a manipulator in the uterus to stand it up and hold the ovaries up. If this isn't done, everything fills the pelvis, and you can't get a proper view. Needless to say, the physician must be thorough and meticulous in searching the entire pelvis for endometriosis.

The fact that so many of my patients have had their experiences with pain ignored or dismissed can be a real problem from a medical standpoint. If the endo is left untreated, not only does a woman have to live with unnecessary pain, the endometriosis will get worse, as

24   Kang SB, Chung HH, Lee JY, Chang YS. Impact of diagnostic laparoscopy on the management of chronic pelvic pain. *Surgical Endoscopy.* 2007;21(6):916-919.

25   Hebbar S, Chawla C. Role of laparoscopy in evaluation of chronic pelvic pain. *Journal of Minimal Access Surgery.* 2005;1(3):116-120.

26   Vercellini P, Fedele L, Arcaini L, Bianchi S, Rognoni MT, Candiani GB. Laparoscopy in the diagnosis of chronic pelvic pain in adolescent women. *Journal of Reproductive Medicine.* 1989;34(10):827-830.

27   Kontoravdis A, Chryssikopoulos A, Hassiakos D, Liapis A, Zourlas PA. The diagnostic value of laparoscopy in 2365 patients with acute and chronic pelvic pain. *International Journal of Gynecology and Obstetrics.* 1996;52(3):243-248.

will the pain. The nervous system can actually start sending out pain signals when it shouldn't or magnifying the intensity of the pain signal. These conditions are known as neuropathic pain and centralization of pain. The more severe the pain and the longer the pain is present, the more these conditions tend to occur. Once they do, it can be difficult, even with surgery, to restore a patient to feeling pain free.

It's very disheartening to hear all the stories my patients tell me about being misdiagnosed. As I've mentioned, I believe treating endometriosis should be its own specialty. Until then, since endo affects so many systems in the body, physicians in other specialties should be more aware of its symptoms and how to treat the disease.

✿ ✿ ✿

"When I was 15, I had eight pelvic exams in five days. After the eighth, I was diagnosed with a polycystic ovary, and the doctor put me on hormones, which may have worsened the cause of my pain, which was endometriosis. Another doctor gave me Vicodin for my pain and suspected interstitial cystitis, but I wasn't referred to any specialists. It wasn't until I did research on my own that I identified the problem as endometriosis." —Lillyth

"The emergency room doctors would rule out appendicitis and gallstones and give me some pain medication. At one ER visit, I was actually told maybe I just had really bad gas. I repeatedly requested a surgical consult, only to be denied. My gynecologist guessed diverticulitis. Wrong. My gastroenterologist was stumped." —Elizabeth

"One doctor referred me to a specialist, who diagnosed me with pelvic inflammatory disease and accused my husband of cheating on me. As it turned out, my husband was faithful, and I did not have PID." —I-Li

"At one hospital, I was diagnosed with irritable bowel syndrome. I wanted to see a gynecologist, but the gastroenterologist thought that was unnecessary. When he examined me, I screamed in pain. He said, 'You are awfully dramatic—this is not supposed to hurt.' Because it was so hard to eat, I lived on juice. Then I was told I was anorexic."
—Lisa

"I've had doctors say I'm a hypochondriac, even when I pointed out that my mother had endometriosis. Sometimes I've wished people could see the mess inside and understand why I'm in pain." —Shannon

Is There a Cure?

Right now there is no definite cure for endometriosis. That doesn't mean patients can't get treatment that offers them relief and allows them to lead normal, active lives. Many if not most women who have endometriosis will not have a recurrence if they get proper treatment.

I think it's useful to compare endometriosis with breast cancer. Both diseases affect millions of women. I think all physicians would agree that while we do not have a cure for breast cancer, we have treatment that's so effective most patients will not have a recurrence. According to the American Cancer Society, the overall survival rates for women diagnosed with breast cancer are 89 percent 5 years after diagnosis, 82 percent after 10 years, and 75 percent after 15 years.[28] Still, we can't tell a breast cancer patient at the end of her treatment that she is "cured."

A good percentage of endometriosis patients will likewise be disease free at 5, 10, or 15 years.[29] Unfortunately, there is no chemotherapy

---

28 American Cancer Society, Breast Cancer Facts & Figures 2009-2010, Atlanta: American Cancer Society, Inc. http://www.cancer.org/acs/groups/content/@nho/documents/document/f861009final90809pdf.pdf. Accessed June 12, 2011.

29 Shakiba K, Bena JF, McGill KM, Minger J, Falcone T. Surgical treatment of endometriosis: a 7-year follow-up on the requirement for further surgery. *Obstetrics and Gynecology.* 2008;111(6):1285-1292.

for endometriosis; it can only be removed surgically. But just as with cancer, if endometriosis is treated correctly, the chance of recurrence is lessened. It largely depends on the skill of the surgeon, but also on other factors: genetics, overall health, age, lifestyle, and nutrition, to name a few. Both endometriosis and breast cancer require a comprehensive, philosophical approach to treatment. That means your doctor should spend the necessary time to talk with you about all aspects of your health, including your diet and the nature of your pain.

So, while there is no guaranteed, 100 percent cure for endo, we can say with confidence that there is effective treatment. When treated appropriately, a significant number of women will regain their health and not suffer from this disease again.

✿ ✿ ✿

"I've had a total of 11 surgeries. My last surgery was in July 2008. There was barely any endometriosis left. Pain, anxiety, and fear no longer control my life." —Elizabeth

"My integrative surgery took place in February 2000, with a team of surgeons. For six hours, they worked on getting rid of my disease for good. Endometriosis was found on my bowels, uterus, and entire pelvic area. After months of recuperation, I was pain free, with no more endometriosis. I could enjoy the simplest things. I could leave my house anytime, even during my periods. I could use the bathroom with no fear or pain. I didn't have to take pain pills. I felt energetic and started exercising at the gym again! February 2010 was my 10-year anniversary of no more endometriosis." —Michele

"I had pain in the scar tissue from a C-section. I went to the original docs who had done the C-section, and they told me I was fine; it was probably just ovulation. It got worse, and I found my present doctor, and he said it was probable that it was endo, and they wouldn't know until they looked.

He did laparoscopic surgery and found that I had all sorts of adhesions and a couple of small hernias, and that my uterus had fused with my abdomen. I recovered, but maybe six or eight months later, I was still having a lot of pain. I went back about a year later, and since he'd already gone in and cleaned everything up, the only thing left was to open up the C-section scar. Sure enough, they found all sorts of endo in the tissue between my skin and muscle. After the second surgery, I've been fantastic. I haven't had any pain; it's been a complete recovery." —Keala

CHAPTER THREE

Myths and Misunderstandings about Endometriosis

Before we go any further, I'd like to clear up some of the many common myths and misunderstandings about this disease.

Causes Myths

Endometriosis can be prevented.

Unfortunately, there's nothing a woman can do to prevent endometriosis. It isn't a disease that's caused by anything a patient did. It's not contagious. As I mentioned earlier, the disease does seem to run in families, and you can't help what you inherit. Some sort of autoimmune response may be triggered that is related to the disease, but at the moment, we don't know much about that. As with any chronic disease of unknown origin, doing everything possible to live a healthy lifestyle will help your body be in the best position to fight off or minimize the severity of the disease.

You can "catch" endometriosis from someone else, from sexual activity, or from a toilet seat.

No, endometriosis cannot be spread from one person to another. While the cause of endo isn't known for sure, we do know that it is not an infectious disease.

Endometriosis can be caused by sexually transmitted diseases.

No, it cannot be transmitted sexually. Endo is often misdiagnosed as pelvic inflammatory disease, which is caused by sexually transmitted diseases, but endo itself is not related to STDs.

Tampons can cause endometriosis.

While there may be a connection between endometriosis and chemicals in the environment, there's no evidence that the chemicals in tampons, which are often bleached, contribute to the disease. On the other hand, it can't hurt to buy chlorine-free tampons, along with organic food, to lessen the chemical load your body has to carry.

Psychological Myths

Women who complain of pain with sex are just having intimacy issues.

Look, if a man complained of pain with sex—pain so severe he felt as if his testicles were being hit repeatedly—would people accuse him of having "intimacy issues"? I don't think so. The pain is all too real. Many women love their significant others so much they are willing to endure hours or days of pain so that they can be intimate.

A history of sexual abuse can cause severe pelvic pain.

There's a widespread belief that women with a history of sexual abuse who experience severe pelvic pain are blowing the pain out of proportion because of unresolved emotional trauma. Sexual abuse does not cause endometriosis or pelvic pain. Of course, a woman who has such a history who also has endometriosis may have to deal with emotional issues surrounding sex and pain. But the pain is caused by the disease.

The pain is all in your head.

No. The pain is in your pelvis, which is located down by your pubic bone. It's not in your head, which is above your shoulders. Nothing could be more frustrating for a woman who is seriously hurting than to be told that she is not really in pain. You know when you're in pain.

Most women who complain of pelvic pain are exaggerating their symptoms.

Sadly, the opposite is true: women with endo often underplay the severity of their symptoms, because they think people won't believe them. But the pain is often more severe than most of us can imagine. Women with endo aren't chronic complainers; they're courageous. In my experience, most of these women push through the pain to do their work and take care of their children, spouse, and significant others. They do everything they can to get up in the morning and forge ahead under the most challenging of circumstances.

Pain and Symptoms Myths

Endometriosis is easy to diagnose because it is the only cause of severe period pain.

It's true that severe pain during periods is a common symptom of endometriosis, but cyclic pain can also be caused by several other conditions, such as ovarian cysts, interstitial cystitis, adhesions, and pelvic varicosities. Hormonal fluctuations and their effects on pain can make some conditions we don't think of as cyclic worse during a woman's period. But when the pain is severe and worsens over time, and when there is pain during intercourse and/or with bowel movements, I suspect endo. While I can usually tell whether a woman has endo from listening to her, doing an exam, and understanding her symptoms, the only way to know for sure is through laparoscopic surgery.

Severe periods during teenage years are normal.

Severe periods are never normal. Some research shows that up to two-thirds of women who suffer from endo had symptoms before they were 20 years old. Girls who begin experiencing acutely painful periods may have already developed endometriosis. Families and physicians should never believe that a girl's pain is exaggerated or normal: if a girl's pain is severe enough to keep her away from school or from participating in sports and day-to-day activities, it's time to find a physician who understands endometriosis and can help her. It can be particularly important to seek out a specialist early on, to ensure that the girls are not traumatized by having their symptoms invalidated, undergoing numerous painful medical tests, or taking ineffective medications with severe side effects, as well as to make sure they get relief from their suffering. If it is not endo, the pain is still serious and needs to be treated.

The symptoms of endometriosis always start in the teen years.

While endo often begins in the teen years, the symptoms can also develop later.

Endometriosis is only painful when you have your period.

In the early stages of endo, pain is worst during the menstrual period. As the disease progresses, however, many women suffer pain throughout the month. It may be worst during their periods, but it may be more debilitating at other times, depending on the activities they do. In the worst cases, women rarely feel relief from the pain.

The more serious the endometriosis, the more severe the pain.

Oddly, this isn't true. Some women can have a lot of endometriosis and little or no pain. Some may have a relatively mild case but experience severe pain because of where the endometriosis is located. But "serious" is a relative term. Any woman who has excruciating pain has a serious case of endometriosis.

You don't have to treat endometriosis with serious pain drugs; over-the-counter medications should be just fine.

Anyone who believes you can treat the severe pain of endo with a little ibuprofen obviously hasn't experienced the pain and has never met someone who has. The pain women experience with endometriosis can be harder to endure than that experienced with surgery or childbirth. In my opinion, it is not humane to withhold treatment, including narcotics, for pain. Wouldn't it seem wrong and unjust to perform surgery without anesthesia or refuse to provide pain relief during childbirth? The fact is, women with endo often need narcotics. Their pain management, of course, needs to be strictly monitored by physicians who can provide the correct combination and dose of medication, along with a comprehensive, longer-term plan to deal with the pain.

If left untreated, endometriosis will continue to spread, and the pain will get worse.

This is often the case, but not always. It's important to remember that endometriosis varies with every patient. You can't predict whether the disease will get worse. But if a woman is already suffering from severe pain and has a history of the disease getting worse, you know it's not going to get better, and it's long past time for appropriate treatment. Endometriosis starts as regular, or nociceptive, pain. If left untreated, it can become neuropathic pain or centralized pain, which are essentially caused by an overloaded and "broken" nervous system. Once that type of pain occurs, it does not go away even after the endo is treated.

Statistics and Facts Myths

You shouldn't have sexual intercourse if you have endometriosis; that can make it worse.

Having sex won't make endo worse, but it can make it more painful. If you are experiencing a lot of pain with sex, you might want to experiment with positions and techniques that will make it less painful and more pleasurable. But if endometriosis is causing difficulties in your sex life, it could be a good idea to seek comprehensive treatment to fix and recover from the problem. That might include surgery, finding a specialized physical therapist to treat pelvic-floor muscle spasm, even consultations with a sex therapist.

Endometriosis invariably causes infertility or sterility.

Many women who have endometriosis are afraid they may never get pregnant. Young women are sometimes told that if they want to have children, they need to get pregnant right away. For those currently not trying to get pregnant, they are often told to postpone surgery.

The misunderstanding behind this recommendation is the belief that fertility is increased only during the first year after surgical removal of endometriosis. This is absolutely false. If the surgery is done properly it will help increase the chances of getting pregnant for many years after the surgery—not just the first year. Because most women with infertility try to get pregnant soon after the endometriosis is removed, an inaccurate association has developed between the time of pregnancy and the removal of the endometriosis. Simply put, once the endometriosis is removed, a woman will be more likely to become pregnant once she tries, assuming no other factors are affecting her fertility. It does not matter if the first attempts are within the first year after surgery or 2nd, 3rd, 4th year, etc, after surgery. Early surgical intervention can also prevent the scarring and damage to the reproductive organs that occur in the more advanced and aggressive forms of Stage III and Stage IV endometriosis. (See page 125 for a more detailed discussion of the stages of endometriosis.)

Overall, endometriosis will decrease the chances of getting pregnant in any given month. But the vast majority of women with endometriosis are able to become pregnant. Some patients with endometriosis become pregnant without any difficulty. Others may require fertility treatment, sometimes including in vitro fertilization. Only a small percentage of women will not be able to conceive. The age of the woman and the egg quality are paramount. For all women, it is best to get pregnant before the age of 35, and especially before the age of 40. Pregnancy can and does happen after the age of 40, but there is a much lower chance of success.

Endometriosis always comes back.
Many if not most women who have proper surgery (laparoscopic surgery with wide excision) will not have a recurrence of the disease. Most cases of rapid recurrence are really the persistence and regrowth of the disease, because some of the endometriosis, which is difficult to see and can be microscopic, was not removed. (See chapter six for more information on surgery.) Most of my patients, after proper

surgery, have found they can resume normal lives; many find that all their pain has disappeared.

Endometriosis leads to cancer.

Endometriosis acts like cancer, invading normal tissue, but it is not a malignancy. It is a benign tumor. (Physicians call these "benign" tumors, but for a woman with endo, they feel anything but benign!) Endometriosis is not a type of cancer, nor is there much good evidence that endo is related to cancer. One Swedish study of more than 63,000 women with endometriosis looked at their risk of cancer and found that overall, their cancer risk was the same as for women who don't have endo. The researchers found a very slightly increased risk for some rare types of cancer, including ovarian cancer, endocrine tumors, kidney cancer, and thyroid cancer. Women with endo actually showed a lower risk of getting cervical cancer. In any case, the increased risk is very small. But it may be another reason to get rid of the atypical cells and growths via surgery.[30]

I personally believe that if left untreated, aggressive forms of Stage IV endometriosis may result in an increased risk of cancer. One study published in the New England Journal of Medicine isolated a genetic mutation that seems to link two types of ovarian cancer with endometriosis, although the researchers pointed out that while women with endo are at a slightly higher risk of developing these cancers, the risk for any individual woman with endometriosis is still very low.[31]

Endometriosis affects only white, professional women who delay childbearing.

No, women of all ages and ethnicities develop endometriosis. Whether a woman chooses to become a mother or not does not have any impact on whether she will get the disease. Endo probably got the reputation as a white woman's disease because it was initially more frequently diagnosed among women with means, who could afford to visit enough

---

30 Melin A, Sparen P, Bergqvist A. The risk of cancer and the role of parity among women with endometriosis. *Human Reproduction*. 2007;22(11):3021-3026.

31 Wiegand KC, Shah SP, Al-Agha OM, et al. ARID1A mutations in endometriosis-associated ovarian carcinomas. *New England Journal of Medicine*. 2010;363(16):1532-1543.

doctors to get a correct diagnosis. Now, however, we know that endo is a worldwide problem, affecting millions of women. Personally, I have great concern for the women in countries that lack access to proper treatment for endometriosis.

Endometriosis is a rare disease.
Endometriosis is not at all rare—it's just not always diagnosed and treated properly. Endo affects more than 5.5 million women in North America; it's estimated that between 2 and 10 percent of American women of childbearing age have the disease. That makes endometriosis more common than many forms of cancer.

Treatments and Cures Myths

The drug Lupron cures endometriosis.
If Lupron, one of a group of drugs known as GnRH agonists, cured endometriosis, life would be much simpler for women suffering from this disease (and for their physicians). But Lupron, used as a first line of defense by some physicians, does not cure endo. Lupron affects brain chemistry by turning off estrogen production by the ovaries and immediately throwing the woman into menopause, with all its side effects. Too many physicians mistakenly think if you take away the estrogen, the endo will die. But studies have shown that the actual endometriosis implants can create their own estrogen, which Lupron doesn't touch; only surgery can do that. The side effects of Lupron can be severe, even worse than the pain it is trying to treat. The benefit of the treatment should always be greater than the side effects. Some physicians have found that the use of "add-back therapy"—giving low doses of estrogen and/or progesterone—help to minimize these side effects. I'm not saying that Lupron will never be helpful, but it is too often misused. All too frequently, patients are being told they will be dismissed from their doctors care if they do not take the Lupron.

If a patient continues to have pain on Lupron, she doesn't have endometriosis.
In the more than 20 years that I have been treating endometriosis, I have met many patients who had been placed on Lupron, did not get

better, and came to me for surgery while still taking the drug. I have almost always found active endometriosis, confirmed by pathology, despite the Lupron. I remember when I was a resident, an attending physician told me, "We will give her Lupron, and if the pain does not go away, that means it's not endo, and we will refer her to another doctor." We now know that's not true. Unfortunately, many physicians still use this approach. I imagine some of their patients are sitting in a psychiatrist's office at this moment.

Hormonal treatments can cure endo.

Drugs based on synthetic hormones, like the Pill, Depo-Provera, Danazol, and Lupron, are used to treat endometriosis. But in most cases, these hormonal treatments just quiet the symptoms, by slowing down the load of estrogen that feeds endo. They usually don't provide long-term relief and can't rid the body of the disease. Only surgery (performed correctly) can do that.

Pregnancy cures endometriosis.

Pregnancy can quiet the symptoms of endo, just as hormonal drug treatments can. But it doesn't make the disease go away. We're not sure why pregnancy helps suppress the disease—perhaps because of changes in the immune system, and/or perhaps because women aren't menstruating during pregnancy and so have no painful periods. Similarly, breastfeeding slows the symptoms of endometriosis because it stops periods. (Breastfeeding inhibits the release of estrogen by the ovaries, so there's less estrogen to feed the endometriosis implants.) Some women, however, experience a worsening of symptoms during pregnancy, which may be related to the stretching and pulling of the endometriosis implants in and around the uterus in the first three months. Most women will find that any beneficial effects of pregnancy on endo are temporary, and they will experience a recurrence when their menstrual periods resume.

Hysterectomy cures endo, and if you have pain after a hysterectomy, you don't have endometriosis.

Hysterectomy alone, with or without removal of the ovaries, is not an appropriate treatment for endometriosis. The endometriosis tissue grows under the ovaries, on the ovaries, on the bowel or bladder, next to the uterus, but rarely right on the uterus. Removing the uterus will leave the disease behind. Some people believe that if the ovaries are removed, too, that will cure the endo, since the ovaries are where the estrogen is coming from. But as we have seen, endometriosis can produce its own estrogen. And removal of the ovaries can result in osteoporosis and a dramatic drop in a woman's sex drive, because the ovaries produce testosterone as well as estrogen.

Since endometrial implants create their own estrogen, they can continue to grow even after a hysterectomy. What happens too often with hysterectomies is that the physician takes the uterus out and leaves the disease, believing that any remaining endo will "melt away." It will not just melt away. It must be cut out and removed from the body. In some patients, especially if they have severe pelvic congestion—adenomyosis—which is endometriosis that has invaded the muscle wall of the uterus, it may be appropriate to perform a hysterectomy to remove all the endometriosis.

Endometriosis goes away with menopause.

Many women may feel relief from their symptoms when they hit menopause in their late forties or early fifties. But endometriosis has been diagnosed in women as late as in their seventies. Menopause stops the flow of estrogen that feeds the endometrial implants, but—just as we've seen with Lupron and hysterectomy—the endometriosis can still produce estrogen. If the endometriosis has caused scarring that is causing pain, menopause will most likely not stop the pain. Again, only surgery can do that.

Any OB/GYN can treat endometriosis.

Surgical treatment of endometriosis requires very specialized techniques that are not taught in the standard OB/GYN residency. In addition, patients often require treatment of various other conditions that the routine OB/GYN physician is not familiar with. Most endometriosis specialists have devoted their lives to treating endometriosis and are advanced laparoscopic surgeons, often with one to three years of extra training after a standard OB/GYN residency. It is appropriate for an OB/GYN to do his or her best to help patients with endometriosis and pelvic pain. The initial step of prescribing birth control pills often works in mild cases. But when the patient is not getting relief, it's best to refer her to a doctor who has extensive experience treating endo with laparoscopic surgery.

I can cure my endometriosis with diet, nutritional supplements, exercise, and acupuncture.

I'm all in favor of complementary therapies, and recommend that all my patients get the exercise and nutritional support they need. There's no doubt that a healthy lifestyle and techniques such as meditation, which support the mind-body connection, will help you feel better and will act synergistically to help your other treatments work better. Acupuncture may relieve some of the pain symptoms. But these techniques alone won't make the disease disappear. If you come across anyone claiming to have a simple herbal cure for endo or selling potions or pills purported to do so (as tempting as they might sound), run in the other direction.

If I have extensive endometriosis that affects my bowels, I'll have to have a bowel resection and wear a colostomy bag.

Sometimes, with severe endo that invades all the way through the bowel wall, the surgeon will have to cut a piece of the bowel out. Many patients are told by their doctors that if they have a bowel resection, they will have to wear a colostomy bag. This is just not true. After we remove the diseased section of the bowel, we put the bowel back together. Besides, as I jokingly tell my patients, it's too hard to find shoes to match a colostomy bag! I wouldn't do that to them.

CHAPTER FOUR

A Healing Relationship: Finding Good Care and Treatment for Endometriosis

Endometriosis is a tricky disease—hard to diagnose and to treat—which is why it is so often overlooked, misdiagnosed, and undertreated. Yet endometriosis is so debilitating, it is the third leading cause of hospitalization for gynecologic reasons in the United States.[32] In the US each year, more than 50,000 women between the ages of 15 and 64 are hospitalized for endometriosis, and at least 5.5 million women are affected at any one time.[33]

As I've said previously, most women with the condition suffer without treatment for years, and when they do get treatment, it is often inadequate. It's shocking to think that worldwide, the average delay in diagnosing the disease is 6 to 11 years—vital, productive years when a woman shouldn't have to live in pain.[34] This chapter is about how you (or your daughter or partner) can finally find effective—and respectful—treatment for endometriosis.

To reiterate, the main symptoms of endo are pelvic pain, difficulties getting pregnant, pain with sexual intercourse (the medical term

---

32 McLeod BS, Retzloff MG. Epidemiology of endometriosis: an assessment of risk factors. *Clinical Obstetrics and Gynecology*. 2010;53(2):389-396.

33 Matalliotakis IM, Cakmak H, Fragouli YG, Goumenou AG, Mahutte NG, Arici A. Epidemiological characteristics in women with and without endometriosis in the Yale series. *Archives of Gynecology and Obstetrics*. 2008;277(5):389–393.

34 McLeod BS, Retzloff MG. Epidemiology of endometriosis: an assessment of risk factors. *Clinical Obstetrics and Gynecology*. 2010;53(2):389-396.

for this is dyspareunia), and cyclic pain that increases in intensity over time. About one-third of patients who suffer chronic pelvic pain, particularly associated with infertility, have endometriosis.[35] If you are experiencing pelvic pain, especially if it interferes with your day-to-day life, you need to see a physician who is experienced in treating this disease. Even if the cause of the pain isn't endometriosis, it is likely a condition that needs to be addressed.

From an epidemiological point of view—that is to say, viewing the increased risk in large populations—other clues that you may have a greater chance of developing endometriosis are if you started your period relatively early, if you have short menstrual cycles (fewer than 27 days), or if you experience a long menstrual flow. Studies have shown that women who eat a lot of red meat,[36] as well as those who are tall[37] and/or redheaded,[38] also have an increased risk of developing the disease. (I know, you can cut down on red meat, but there's not much you can do about your height or natural hair color!)

The biggest risk factor is having family members who have endometriosis; studies report that women whose sisters or mothers have had endometriosis have a 4 to 11 times greater risk of getting the disease.[39] Remember, epidemiology looks at large groups, not individuals: having red hair doesn't mean you're going to develop endometriosis. It's just that studies indicate you might have a slightly elevated risk of getting it. Be sure to let your doctor know of any family history of

---

35 Pauerstein CJ. Clinical presentation and diagnosis. In: Schenken RS, ed. *Endometriosis: Contemporary Concepts in Clinical Management*. Philadelphia, PA: JB Lippincott; 1989:127-144.

36 Parazzini F, Chiaffarino F, Surace M, Chatenoud L, Cipriani S, Chiantera V, Benzi G, Fedele L. Selected food intake and risk of endometriosis. *Human Reproduction*. 2004;19(8):1755–1759.

37 Hedgier ML, Hartnett HJ, Louis GM. Association of endometriosis with body size and figure. *Fertility and Sterility*, 2005;84(5):1366–1374.

38 Missmer SA, Spiegelman D, Hankinson SE, Malspeis S, Berbieri RL, Hunter DJ. Natural hair color and the incidence of endometriosis. *Fertility and Sterility*. 2006;85(4):866–870.

39 Matalliotakis IM, Arici A, Cakmak H, Goumenou AG, Koumantakis G, Mahutte NG. Familial aggregation of endometriosis in the Yale Series. *Archives of Gynecology and Obstetrics*. 2008;278(6):507–511.

endometriosis, as well as details about when you started menstruating and how long your period usually lasts.

Whatever your risk factors for endometriosis, the bottom line is that if you have serious pelvic pain, you need to get some seriously good care.

Advocating for Your Health

If you suspect you have endo, you'll have to make it a priority to find the best care possible. Bear in mind that not all OB/GYNs are well informed about this disease. You'll want to get a referral to a doctor who has experience with endometriosis and years of laparoscopic surgery under his or her belt. Because endo usually involves several other physical problems, you'll want to find a doctor who will consider the entire state of your health, not just the endometriosis. Unfortunately, it may not be easy to find such a physician. I see women in my office every single week who have been misdiagnosed; others who have been correctly diagnosed but put on inappropriate medications; still others who have had unsuccessful surgeries.

If you have or suspect you have endometriosis, you will have to be proactive about your medical care. You should learn as much as you can about this disease, so that you can understand your treatment options. You may have to fight with your insurance provider; you may have to travel; you may have to pay more out of pocket than you expected. But you've got to make sure you get good care, and you can't give up until you do. No matter what any physician says to you, you have to trust yourself. It's your body, and you know when you're in pain and when you feel right.

There are many very good OB/GYNs out there, but in the current medical environment, few have the time or skills to get to the bottom of a difficult case of endometriosis. It's a lot easier and cheaper to give patients pills or shots, even when surgery is indicated. It's easier to do a quick hysterectomy than to patiently root out the endometriosis. It isn't uncommon for doctors to clean out the obvious endo and leave some behind, either because they don't have the experience to recognize all the different types of endometriosis or because they lack the skill or time to make sure all the endo is gone.

But good treatment exists, and you should be an advocate for yourself and push for it. In the age of the Internet, a lot of information is available to you, as are informed women in endometriosis chat groups who can relate to your symptoms and help you. (See the Resources section at the end of this book, especially Endometriosis Support Groups.)

Characteristics of a Healing Relationship

Too often, physician-patient relationships look like parent-child interactions. Physicians adopt a paternalistic attitude, and patients feel condescended to. They feel they're not being listened to, that all the power is in the physician's hands. The sad fact is that too often, physicians really *aren't* fully listening to their patients. They have many other patients to see; they may feel helpless treating a complicated disease they don't understand well; and, of course, everyone is always watching the clock and costs, often to the detriment of good care.

But the only way to have a good healing relationship is if your physician treats you like an adult and listens to you with respect. I believe treating endometriosis has to be a partnership. My patients are making big decisions, and often there's no easy answer as to whether they should, for instance, have a hysterectomy or not. I can guide a patient, but ultimately it's her decision as to which treatment option is best for her. I encourage my patients to bring their spouses or significant others to our appointments, because their participation is important in coping with the disease—understanding the suffering their loved one faces and validating the pain she's experiencing—and aiding in the healing process.

Traditionally, physicians have had a mechanical view of the human body: they focus on one problem and ignore its relationship to the rest of the body, particularly the mind. Surgeons might as well be fixing cars or plumbing. But we know that any disease resonates throughout the body; it is affected by attitude, spirit, nutrition, and the interplay of other systems in the body. If you trust your doctor and feel you're in good hands, that attitude will bring you more success in getting healthy.

I may sound idealistic about the kind of doctor-patient relationship I advocate, and I know it may not be possible for all doctors in the current cost-conscious medical environment. But several studies support the notion that a respectful approach to healing is most effective.

From a medical point of view, *healing* means that the patient is cured when possible, and that his or her suffering is reduced when it is not. In one study, after researchers interviewed clinicians who had been successful healers, as well as patients who said they had experienced positive healing relationships, a pattern emerged. Here are the three most important characteristics of a good healing relationship:[40]

- *Valuing* Physicians who can create an emotional bond with patients do so by being nonjudgmental, empathetic, and fully present—not distracted, dismissive, or critical. The patient feels listened to, respected, and valued.

- *Appreciating power* A good healer recognizes that the clinician-patient relationship is inherently asymmetrical—the physician has more power and knowledge in medical matters—and consciously manages his or her power in ways that most benefit the patient. The physician communicates directly to the patient in language she understands, not medical jargon. He or she doesn't leave procedures and treatments mysterious but clarifies them. Sometimes a physician needs to be more of a coach, pushing and encouraging the patient to follow treatment recommendations and take good care of her health. But it's always best when physician and patient can act in partnership.

---

40 Scott JG, Cohen D, di Cicco-Bloom B, Miller WL, Stange KC, Crabtree BF. Understanding healing relationships in primary care. *Annals of Family Medicine*. 2008;6(4):315-322.

- *Abiding* Abiding refers to the physician's care over time, showing commitment to the patient—for instance, returning phone calls—and letting the patient know she will not be abandoned. When patients know their doctors are there for them, they relax and trust in both doctor and treatment.

The researchers found that when the healing relationship had these three components, the outcomes for patients were trust, hope, and a sense of being "known."

Trust means the patient is willing to be vulnerable, to describe symptoms that may be embarrassing or have caused her to feel unwarranted shame. This is crucial. With endometriosis, you have to be able to talk about the most intimate matters: your sex life, your periods, your pain. Trust is knowing that your doctor will do his or her best to take care of you, and that promises will be kept. This is very, very different from the experiences of patients I've seen who have told me they've felt their best bet was to lie, so that the doctor didn't think they were chronic complainers, hypochondriacs, or looking for drugs.

Hope is the belief that a positive future lies beyond the present suffering. Instead of making the rounds from one doctor to another and getting no relief, thinking you'll live with chronic pain that will only get worse, you believe that your pain will go away and you'll be back to doing the things you love: walking freely, bicycling, making plans, meeting friends, being intimate with your partner. No one should be told that she is "just going to have to live with this."

Being known is the sense that the clinician has come to know you beyond what he or she reads on the chart, that he or she "gets" who you are, not to mention what you've been through. Being known is a very positive, comforting feeling that helps a patient believe that she's in a true partnership toward better health.

I realize it's not easy to find a physician like this, but it's important to try, because it's going to make a big difference in the quality of your treatment and, ultimately, your life. If your physician sees no alterna-

tive to putting you on Lupron or suggests that nothing further can be
done about your pain, you need to get a second opinion. Or a third.

❁ ❁ ❁

"After a lot of research, I finally found a doctor who put
me at ease. I was never dismissed, and he believed what
I told him. During my first appointment, the examination
was completely different. I was treated with respect, and I
felt relieved." —Lillyth

"I always had faith in the medical community. My father
was a physician, and my mother, a registered nurse. But by
the end of my two-year experience with doctors who misdiagnosed my endo—with endless tests, sonograms, blood
draws, X-rays, stool cultures, endoscopy, barium swallow,
colonoscopy—*doctor* had become a four-letter word. Finally I found a doctor who sent me lengthy questionnaires
and actually wanted to know the patient! He respectfully
and patiently answered each of my many, many questions.
Leaving his office, I felt a glimmer of something I had given
up on: hope." —Elizabeth

"For five years, I went through a series of tests and doctors,
only to be told there was nothing wrong and that tests indicated my condition was normal. I searched on the Internet
and found from a support group that there were many
women struggling just like me. That led me to my doctor.
We scheduled a conference call, and for the first time, I
spoke to a physician who was able to understand and describe exactly what I was feeling. At my appointment, there
was a warm welcome by the doctor and his staff, followed by
three days of extensive tests that included questions about
nutrition, lifestyle, pain tolerance, and more. I came armed
with all the right questions. I traveled across the country for
a six-hour surgery, and after months of recuperation, I am
now pain free with no endometriosis." —Michele

"I got the name of a doctor hundreds of miles away but decided I needed to tackle this problem. I was nervous, afraid of being treated poorly. But I was also fed up and determined. There was a voice inside me that said, 'If this doctor can't help me, I'm going to die.' I had been through too much pain over the past two years. When the doctor entered the room, I started to cry. Through my tears, I answered his questions. He looked at me and said, 'You are not going crazy.' He was very thorough and ordered a lot of tests. I had to have surgery, and I felt anxious. The last step toward good health is faith, and I wanted to have faith. 'Don't worry, Bess, I'm going to help you,' the doctor said before surgery. His reassurance helped. When I awoke, I was pain free." —Bessy

How to Be a Partner in Your Care

You will have a better experience with your physician if you do everything you can to get him or her on board your case. As you know, physicians are pressed for time, so the easier you make their job for them, the more help you're likely to get. Many doctors will send you paperwork before your appointment, so that they'll have a chance to review your history before you get there. Even if your physician doesn't do that, you can save time by being organized.

Come to your appointment with the following items:

- A list of the main issues you want to address
- A list of all the medications you're taking
- A list of the symptoms you're having and when you have them relative to your menstrual cycle
- A list of previous physicians you've seen and procedures you've had
- A list of the top questions you'd like to have answered
- A positive attitude

It is helpful if you know the main issues you want addressed. You may have a lot of symptoms, but you want to focus on what's bothering you most. When your time is up, if all your questions haven't been answered, ask if you can make a follow-up appointment. This shows you respect the physician's time and constraints but want to get the best care possible.

Your attitude is going to help you get the best treatment you can. You want to be informed and proactive, but understand that some physicians feel threatened if you come in acting as if you've learned everything there is to know about endometriosis from the Internet. Respect goes two ways.

How to Find a Good Doctor

This is a complex disease that often does not have clear-cut answers; many different treatment modalities may be needed. It's important to find a physician who takes your condition seriously, is open to various types of treatment, will coordinate care with other doctors, and, of course, has experience in the treatment of endometriosis and pelvic pain. In addition, look for an outstanding surgeon with advanced surgical skills, because most women with endometriosis will need the disease removed surgically.

Treating endometriosis surgically requires much more skill than performing a hysterectomy. Interestingly, only a small minority of OB/GYNs have the necessary surgical skills to perform a laparoscopic hysterectomy. Data from two recent studies shows that only 12 to 14 percent of hysterectomies are performed laparoscopically, while 22 percent are performed vaginally. The vast majority, 64 to 66 percent, are abdominal hysterectomies, performed through a laparotomy, the large "bikini" incision.[41, 42] However, when surveyed, only 8 percent

---

41 Wu JM, Wechter ME, Geller EJ, Nguyen TV, Visco AG. Hysterectomy rates in the United States, 2003. *Obstetrics and Gynecology.* 2007;110(5):1091–1095.

42 Jacoby VL, Autry A, Jacobson G, Domush R, Nakagawa S, Jacoby A. Nationwide use of laparoscopic hysterectomy compared with abdominal and vaginal approaches. *Obstetrics and Gynecology.* 2009;114(5):1041-1048.

of OB/GYN doctors would prefer an abdominal hysterectomy done through a "bikini" incision for themselves or their spouse. When asked why they were not providing their patients with the kind of surgery they themselves would prefer, the most common reasons they gave were lack of training during residency, the technical difficulty of laparoscopic surgery, lack of personal laparoscopic surgical experience, and the longer operating time required by the laparoscopic approach. In response to this data, the editor of the journal in which the surveys were published commented, "Residency programs in the United States continue to provide inadequate training and experience in laparoscopic and vaginal approaches to hysterectomy."[43]

While it is accepted that the majority of hysterectomies are performed through an open "bikini" incision, this is not the case for treating endometriosis. It is expected by both patients and physicians that endometriosis be treated laparoscopically. Yet laparoscopic treatment of endometriosis is far more difficult to do than performing a laparoscopic hysterectomy. If the majority of OB/GYNs do not feel qualified to perform a laparoscopic hysterectomy, how can they treat endometriosis laparoscopically?

If your OB/GYN is one of the 12 percent performing hysterectomies laparoscopically, there's a better chance he or she has the necessary surgical skills to remove your endometriosis. If your OB/GYN is still performing hysterectomies through the large "bikini" incision, keep looking for another doctor. Once you find an endometriosis surgeon who performs laparoscopies, make sure he or she uses wide excision, as opposed to coagulation or cautery. (For more information on these techniques, see pages 94–116.)

Finally, to help in your search for the right doctor for you, here are questions to ask when looking for a doctor and questions to ask yourself after your first meeting.

---

43   Einarsson JI, Matteson KA, Schulkin J, Chavan NR, Sangi-Haghpeykar H. Minimally Invasive hysterectomies – a survey on attitudes and barriers among practicing gynecologists. *Journal of Minimally Invasive Gynecology.* 2010;17(2):167-175.

Before you make an appointment, ask yourself the following questions:

- Does the physician specialize in treating endometriosis? Does the physician have years of experience doing laparoscopic surgery with wide excision? Does the physician use excision and vaporization (the preferred method of laparoscopic surgery) rather than coagulation?

- Does the physician primarily prescribe Lupron or do hysterectomies to treat endometriosis?

- Does the physician work with a team? This might include on-site or referrals to a nurse practitioner, nutritionist, psychologist, mind/body practitioner, physical therapist, urologist, gastroenterologist, and pain-management specialist.

- Have women in support groups or online chat groups for endometriosis had good experiences with this doctor?

After you meet with the physician, ask yourself the following questions:

- Did your doctor show that he or she cared about you as a person and would be there when needed? Did the doctor and the staff show respect and abiding interest by returning your phone calls, not rushing you through your appointment, and taking your concerns seriously? Did the doctor thoroughly explain your treatment options?

- Did you feel that you were treated as an adult and listened to with respect? Did the physician take the time to take a thorough medical history and ask about your diet, exercise, and lifestyle?

- Did the physician suggest that your significant other attend the appointments?

- Did the doctor respect complementary therapies, such as acupuncture and meditation, rather than dismissing them out of hand?

PART II
Diagnosis
AND Treatment
of Endometriosis, Pelvic Pain,
and Associated Conditions

CHAPTER FIVE

Diagnosing Endometriosis and Other Causes of Pelvic Pain

Endometriosis Is Not the Only Cause of Pelvic Pain

Endometriosis is a leading cause of pelvic pain, but it is not the only cause of pelvic pain. While it is important to properly diagnose and treat endo, it is also important not to overlook other factors contributing to the patient's pain. I often use the analogy of sitting on thumbtacks: if a person is sitting on one thumbtack, and I take it out, she will feel better. If she is sitting on four or five thumbtacks and I remove one, she will still have significant pain. We need to find and treat as many of the patient's pain generators as possible.

For example, I saw a new patient awhile back who had had surgery for endometriosis and felt it was returning, so she was coming to see me for another surgery. After evaluating her, I thought she might be having pain from food sensitivities—in her case, to wheat or gluten. While her symptoms could have been a result of recurrent endo, I asked if she would be willing to eliminate wheat and gluten from her diet for a couple of weeks. When I saw her about a month later, I asked how she was doing. She said, "Great! I am about 90 percent better!" Needless to say, she did not have recurrent endo and did not need surgery.

Part of the challenge of treating pelvic pain is determining with each patient what is causing the pain, because endometriosis is often present with other conditions that have similar symptoms.

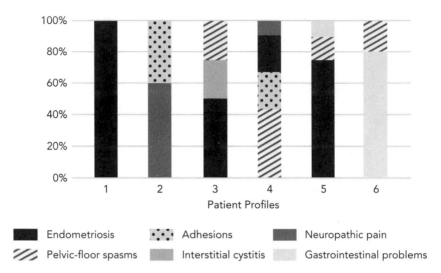

Figure 1. Different Causes of Pelvic Pain

This chart illustrates a few examples of my typical experience, over the years, with patients who come in presenting symptoms of pelvic pain. You can see that there are usually various co-conditions with endo, all of which need to be addressed. Examples of related problems include adhesions (scar tissue), interstitial cystitis (IC), pelvic-floor muscle spasms, neuropathic pain, and gastrointestinal (GI) problems.

Sit Down and Listen to the Patient

Most books and websites about this disease will tell you that endometriosis cannot be diagnosed without looking inside the patient with a laparoscope. Strictly speaking, this is true. Though researchers are working on it, there is no blood test that you can send to a lab, no imaging machine that will take a clear picture of the disease. In one recent study, researchers analyzed 133 different proteins found in the urine of 11 women with endometriosis and 6 women without endometriosis. They found one protein, cytokeratin-19, in much higher concentrations in the women with endometriosis. While it's encouraging to think that a urine test might eventually help us diagnose endo, the study used a very small number of women, and the results are preliminary. Further studies and validation need to take place before this kind of test could become clinically available.[44] To be 100 percent certain it's endo, you have to see it inside the pelvic region. However, when I hear a patient say that she's always had bad periods but they got worse over time, that she has pain with sex and shooting pain in her abdomen, that she feels an awful tugging inside—when I listen to everything she has to say about her condition, I can usually tell if she has endo. After 20 years of treating endometriosis in private practice, I can say that if I had only one test to choose from, I would choose listening to the patient, because that technique is the most accurate. The patient is not a doctor, but she lives with her body and knows what is going on in it.

The Physical Exam

There's more to diagnosis than the crucial step of listening to the patient, of course. After taking a detailed medical history and hearing her story—which can take a couple of hours—I do a physical exam, including a pelvic exam. I want to understand the total picture of my patient's health, not just the symptoms she came in with. Here are a few of the things I look for and why:

- One shoulder higher than the other shows biomechanical misalignment. This can result in stress points that can cause pain. Patients with this problem might benefit from adding physical therapy to their overall treatment plan.

- A swelling in the neck can indicate an enlarged thyroid, which is usually the result of a low-functioning thyroid gland.

- Misalignment of the jaw can cause TMJ (temporomandibular joint disorder) and cranial-sacral problems, which in some patients can contribute to pelvic pain.

---

44 Tokushige N, Markham R, Crossett B, Ahn SB, Nelaturi VL, Khan A, Fraser IS. Discovery of a novel biomarker in the urine in women with endometriosis. *Fertility and Sterility*. 2011;95(1):46-49.

- Pain under the right rib can mean a malfunctioning gall-bladder.

- If the abdominal wall is tender when I push on it, I have the patient do a crunch or sit-up. If the pain is worse, it is most likely from nerve pain in the abdominal wall. If the pain is not worse, the problem is most likely located deep in the abdomen or pelvis (endo pain, bowel pain).

- I push on the bladder to see if it is tender.

- I check the 18 fibromyalgia points for pain.

- I look for pain that would be consistent with a hernia or a problem with the psoas muscle or something else besides endo.

- I even check a patient's dental work to see if she has mercury amalgams. There is some evidence that the mercury can off-gas and adversely affect the patient's health. We don't have a definitive answer as to the real risk of mercury, but we do have more modern, safer alternatives, called composite fillings.

The pelvic exam starts with a Q-tip. There is a small area around the opening of the vagina, called the vestibule, which can hurt even if lightly touched with the Q-tip. This is an indication of a condition separate from endometriosis, vestibulitis, which I will describe later in this chapter. It can cause pain when you are just sitting around, as well as during intercourse, and it affects millions of women.

Next, I check the pelvic-floor muscles, the ones that make up the bottom of the pelvis going from the pubic bone, in the front, to the tailbone, in the back. Just as tension causes many people to get knots in their neck and shoulder muscles, patients with pelvic pain can unconsciously tense their pelvic muscles. Over time, these muscles may start to go into spasm, which can cause excruciating pain.

Then I check the pudendal nerves, which are located halfway up the vagina. When these nerves are damaged, it can cause pudendal neuralgia (nerve pain). After that, I palpate the deep organs, including the bladder, cervix, uterus, and ovaries, to discover any pain or abnormalities. If a patient's pelvis feels frozen, that's a pretty sure sign of advanced Stage III or Stage IV endometriosis. It can mean the bowel is being eaten away by the disease, and the potential for a partial bowel resection. In those cases, I often do a rectal exam, too, to see if I can feel any endo lumps in that region.

Transvaginal Sonogram

After the manual exam, I usually do an ultrasound (also called a transvaginal sonogram) in the pelvis. Using a wand that goes up inside the vagina, I can see the location and position of the uterus, the uterus wall and thickness of the lining, polyps in the uterus, fibroids in the wall of the uterus (adenomyosis) and any abnormality of the uterus. I can see if both ovaries are normal or whether there's a cyst in them. I can usually see an endometrioma, a "chocolate cyst," which is endometriosis in the ovary. I am also looking for varicose veins, endometriosis in the wall of the uterus, and even scar tissue. When I gently push the bowel and uterus, they should roll over each other; if they move together, they are probably stuck together with scar tissue. What I can't see with the sonogram are any small implants of endometriosis peppering the walls of the pelvis.

Some gynecologists have a technician do the sonogram. Then a radiologist looks at the pictures and sends a written report to the ordering physician. I do the sonogram myself, to try to duplicate and locate the pain. It's a kind of pain mapping. As I'm doing the sonogram, I put gentle pressure on different places and ask the patient whether pressure on that spot reproduces her pain. If it does, I'll ask, for instance, if it's some of the deep pain she's told me she's experienced with intercourse. She'll say yes or no, guide me in the right direction—for example, more to the left or right. By talking with my patient as I do the sonogram, I can get a mental picture of what's going on inside her. Once we locate the pain, we can see exactly where it is with the sonogram: the uterus, ovaries, bladder, the area behind the uterus next to the bowel, on the pelvis, under the ovary, or even if it is not in the pelvis.

By listening, doing a manual pelvic exam, and doing a sonogram that maps the pain, I will have a clear idea of whether a patient needs surgery by the end of the first exam. Even if I strongly suspect she has endo, I'll want to know how her other systems are functioning, so we'll run a series of tests, which vary depending on the patient's medical history. If I suspect food allergies, we'll have her do an elimination diet. We'll look at her levels of vitamin D, thyroid functioning, estrogen metabolism, and do other tests that will give me a good picture of her overall health and functioning, as well as eliminate some other possible diseases.

I'll also review reports on the patient's previous operations, if any. This can be crucial in predicting where endometriosis might be deeply buried. Sometimes, finding endo is like digging for buried treasure, and previous operative reports can be a map to help find it once we're in surgery.

Residual Endometriosis—Patient Assisted Laparoscopy (PAL)

When I see a patient who has already had surgery for endometriosis, there's always a possibility that some of the endo has been left inside. This can range from obvious endometriosis the surgeon was not able to remove to deeply buried endometriosis that cannot be seen at laparoscopy.

I had a memorable case like this a couple of years ago. She had been in pain for more than 30 years and had had many surgeries, including a hysterectomy, with some very good endometriosis surgeons. She thought she would have to live with the pain for the rest of her life. I did what is called a patient-assisted laparoscopy, or PAL. I used a tiny fiber-optic laparoscope, about the size of a needle used to draw blood, to poke around inside the patient while she was awake. She was able to tell me the exact location of the pain. In this case, it was a remnant of the ligament attached to the top of the uterus prior to the hysterectomy. It looked completely normal from the surface, with no visible endo, but when I touched it, it consistently reproduced her pain. After the PAL was completed, the patient was given general anesthesia and traditional laparoscopic surgery was begun. As I started to remove it, I saw that it was scarred as far as the blood vessels going down to her leg. Eventually I got all the scar tissue and remnant ligament out. When she woke up from surgery, her pain was gone for the first time in decades. And when I got the lab results from the pathologist, they showed that this "mass of scar tissue" was endometriosis!

Pelvic Pain Not Caused by Endometriosis

It's important to remember that while pelvic pain is the hallmark of endometriosis, not all pelvic pain is caused by endometriosis. Part of the challenge in dealing with pelvic pain is the wide range of medical conditions and traditional medical subspecialties that can be involved, which is one reason why it is so often mistreated and why one condition can be treated while another is overlooked. (Often, the patient is left to coordinate her care from the different physicians and specialties.) There can be many sources of non-endometriosis pain, all of which a doctor needs to consider before doing surgery.

Non-Endometriosis Causes of Pelvic Pain

- Interstitial cystitis
- Pelvic-floor muscle spasm
- Adhesions or scar tissue
- Fibroids
- Adenomyosis
- Uterine retroversion
- Pelvic congestion
- Abdominal-wall neuropathy and pudendal nerve entrapment (PNE)
- Pudendal neuropathy
- Food allergies and food sensitivities
- Ovarian remnant
- Foreign body
- Hernias
- Appendicitis
- Gastrointestinal problems (motility problems, redundant colon, diverticulosis, anal fissure)
- Lyme disease
- Generalized visceral hypersensitivity
- Vulvodynia

Interstitial Cystitis (IC)

Interstitial cystitis, also known as painful bladder syndrome (PBS), is a chronic condition of the bladder that often mimics a bladder infection.

It is estimated that more than four million people in the United States have IC. Interstitial cystitis and endometriosis have been called the evil twins: one doesn't cause the other, but it is not uncommon for both to be present in a patient with pelvic pain.[45, 46] The pain associated with IC can get worse with a woman's periods and can also result in pain with intercourse.

Patients with IC can experience pelvic pain, pelvic pressure, pain during urination, urinary frequency, and urinary urgency. They tend to have smaller bladder capacities and can have glomerulations (small-capillary bleeding from the bladder wall) or Hunner's ulcers (lesions or sores on the lining of the bladder). My new patient-history form includes a Pelvic Pain and Urinary Frequency Questionnaire, also known as the PUF score; a high score highlights the possibility that IC is contributing to the patient's pain. To help make a diagnosis, I often do what is called a cystoscopy with hydrodistention. With this procedure, the bladder is filled with fluid (distended) and examined with a small, lighted tube (cystoscope) inserted up through the urethra under anesthesia.

Unlike endometriosis, IC cannot be removed surgically. It is usually treated with prescription medications or diet modifications. Elmiron is the FDA-approved prescription medication, usually in a dose of 100 mg three times a day. It can take weeks or months for the medication to work; I usually ask patients to take it for three months before giving up on it if it doesn't seem to be working. I also use the prescription drug hydroxyzine, usually 25 mg before bed. (It is somewhat like an antihistamine, so drowsiness can be a side effect.)

With some patients, certain foods will exacerbate the IC symptoms. I recommend that patients keep a journal noting their symptoms and the foods they eat. It can be difficult to determine if a particular food is the problem. The best approach is to stop eating just one type of food for two weeks and then add it back into the diet. If the bladder

---

45   Nazif O, Teichman JM, Gebhart GF. Neural upregulation in interstitial cystitis. *Urology.* 2007;69(4 Suppl):24-33.

46   Berkley KJ. A life of pelvic pain. *Physiology and Behavior.* 2005;86(3):272-280.

symptoms improved for a time, then got worse when the patient began eating that food again, it was probably one of the culprits. This doesn't mean you can never eat that food. If your bladder is doing well, go ahead; but if you are having a rough time, it's probably best to avoid it for a while.

Bladder instillations may be helpful. Here, the bladder is filled with a drug called dimethyl sulfoxide (Rimso-50), or DMSO. When it is retained for about 15 minutes and then expelled, it seems to reduce inflammation and block pain. Two therapies—transcutaneous electrical nerve stimulation (TENS) and interferential therapy, where mild electrical pulses stimulate the nerves to the bladder—may also be used when diet and prescription medications are not effective. Some physicians feel that implanting an Interstim device, an electrical neuromodulator, has helped some IC patients.[47] Physical therapy may be helpful, especially if the bladder pain has resulted in pelvic-floor muscle spasm.

Pelvic-floor Muscle Spasm

Patients with long-standing endometriosis and pelvic pain often develop pelvic-floor muscle spasm. You know how incredible the pain is with this condition if you've ever had a charley horse in your leg. The pain from the spasm in the pelvic-floor muscles, extending from the pubic bone to the tailbone, can be triggered by activity, including sexual intercourse, or can be present 24/7. I often refer these patients to a physical therapist experienced with pelvic-floor therapy, and many have found significant relief. However, most physical therapists do not have training in or treat pelvic-floor muscle spasm, so it is important to find a physical therapist who has had this specific training. (See chapter nine.)

Adhesions or Scar Tissue

Adhesion is the medical term for scar tissue, which is abnormal tissue that can form during the healing process. Scar tissue inside the body

---

47   For more information on interstitial cystitis, see http://www.ichelp.org, or http://kidney. niddk.nih.gov/kudiseases/pubs/interstitialcystitis

often connects two parts of the body that are not supposed to be connected, which, needless to say, can result in pain.

Three basic types of scar tissue, or adhesions, may connect normal body parts. Filmy adhesions are similar to spider webs and don't usually cause pain. Since there are few blood vessels running through this type of adhesion, they easily give way if the surgeon sweeps an instrument through them.

Vascular adhesions are more like thick string or ropes connecting two organs, for example, the ovary to the bowel. Scar tissue that forms after surgery usually does so in the first couple of days or weeks, rarely after months or years. However, this type of adhesion can become shorter as it matures, shrinking and leading to a pulling sensation. For this reason, the pain can become progressively worse in the months following surgery.

Dense cohesive adhesions connect two pieces of tissue tightly, with no space between them, like two pieces of wood glued together. They are the most difficult to remove and the most likely to recur. The most common location in which gynecologists see this type of adhesion is between the ovary and the pelvic sidewall. The patient may experience pain just prior to ovulation, when the follicular cyst forms and tugs on the adhesion.

Scar tissue can also be present without connecting two body parts. This is a tough, leathery type of tissue, such as the thick tissue that can be left after a severe burn. Inside the body, this tissue can cause pain when growing on the nerves, bowel, or ureter (the tube from the kidney to the bladder). Remember, scar tissue tends to shorten over time. When it is growing on normal tissue, it tends to constrict the tissue or restrict its movement, ever tightening its grip. This can result in pressure on a nerve, abnormal bowel motility, or narrowing the ureter, which would cause dilation upstream and pain, usually in the mid-back. The pain can be local, at the site of the adhesions, or remote, as when pelvic adhesions cause pain that radiates down the leg.

Scar tissue should be removed to allow the remaining normal, healthy tissue to heal properly. There are two crucial aspects to getting rid of scar tissue. The first is surgical removal of all the adhesions; the second is preventing them from coming back during the healing process. Remember, adhesions form or re-form in the first couple of days and weeks after surgery. If they are not present a month after surgery, they will not re-form.

Merely cutting the adhesions is not enough, since this will leave scar tissue that can adhere to other tissue again. All of the abnormal adhesive tissue should be completely removed. A laser laparoscope is particularly useful in treating thick and/or cohesive adhesions, helping to minimize trauma to the normal tissue. Laser laparoscopy is ideal for removing the leathery type of tissue that squeezes normal tissue, allowing for the removal of the fibrous scar tissue while leaving the normal tissue unharmed. (See chapter six.)

The single most important factor in preventing adhesions from re-forming is good surgical technique. Even so, once scar tissue has formed, there is always a chance it may form again. If two structures (the ovary and the bowel, say) are touching during the healing process, the body, mistaking the two structures for one, may heal them as one, forming scar tissue around them both.

There is an old saying in medicine, "Once adhesions, always adhesions; do not operate, or you will make them worse." In my experience, this is not true. Adhesions can be treated effectively with good surgical techniques combined with supportive adhesion-prevention products. Though more effective products are in development, several supportive measures are available, to be used at the completion of surgery.

- *Interceed* The most common supportive measure is Interceed, which looks like a white mesh material but turns into a gel once placed via the laparoscope. Interceed acts as a temporary barrier to keep surfaces from sticking together and forming adhesions. After about a week, it dissolves and is eliminated from the body. Studies of patients who received Interceed following their surgeries have indicated a reduction in the amount and degree of adhesion formation. (I was involved in some of the initial studies.) If any oozing (minimal bleeding) is present, however, it appears that Interceed can actually increase the formation of adhesions, an opinion shared by several members of the medical community. When there is no oozing, Interceed seems to be very helpful in reducing adhesions.

- *Seprafilm* This product looks like waxed paper but also turns into a gel once inside the body; it dissolves and is eliminated about a month after surgery. Studies have shown that Seprafilm reduces the number and extent of adhesions. Its primary disadvantage is that it is virtually impossible to place through the laparoscope; it is brittle and fairly difficult to place at laparotomy.

- *Gore-Tex Soft Tissue Patch* The Gore-Tex Soft Tissue Patch (previously Gore-Tex Surgical Membrane), which looks a bit like white plastic paper, was another development in adhesion prevention. I was involved in the first gynecologic studies of the Gore-Tex Surgical Membrane, at Johns Hopkins Hospital with Dr. John Rock and have used it following myomectomy, or surgery to remove fibroids in the uterus. It works well, although fairly large pieces are needed, and they must be sutured into place. The primary disadvantage is that it is a permanent foreign body, which could increase the risk of infection; a second surgery may be needed to remove it.

- *ADEPT* ADEPT® Adhesion Reduction Solution was approved by the FDA in August 2006. Its use is indicated for the reduction of postsurgical adhesions in patients having adhesions removed during laparoscopy.

- *SprayShield* This "adhesion barrier system" offers surgeons a unique synthetic, sprayable hydrogel that provides a strong barrier between tissue and organ planes, helping to reduce the development of postsurgical adhesions. Its use is indicated for both open and laparoscopic abdominopelvic surgical procedures. It was released for use in

Europe in October 2008 but is not yet available in the United States.

- *Adhibit* This is also a synthetic hydrogel, sprayed onto the surgical site as two separate streams of polyethylene glycol-based precursor liquids. These rapidly cross-link on the target tissue to form a flexible, adherent, bioabsorbable gel barrier. Adhibit is chemically identical to Angiotech's CoSeal® surgical compound. I have used it in a lab and feel that it holds promise; in fact, several years ago Vital Health Institute was slated to be one of the study centers for clinical trials. However, the FDA is requiring manufacturers to demonstrate that anti-adhesion products demonstrate a reduction of pain as well. Although it has been approved in Europe, to prevent or reduce postsurgical adhesion formation in pediatric patients undergoing cardiac surgery, Adhibit has not been approved for sale in the United States.

Fibroids

Many women have fibroids (benign tumors) in their uterus, but no pain or other symptoms. If they are symptomatic—causing bleeding, pressure, or pain—treatment may be necessary. About one-third of all women develop fibroid tumors within the wall of the uterus. If you have a feeling of pressure in the pelvis, which can cause frequent urination and pain during intercourse, you may have a large fibroid tumor or possibly many smaller fibroid tumors.

Usually, fibroids can be removed either laparoscopically or hysteroscopically (via the cervix) with minimally invasive surgery, especially if they are not so big that they fill the abdomen higher than the belly button. The most common procedure is a myomectomy, which removes the fibroid while preserving the uterus. In some cases, a woman may elect to have a laparoscopic hysterectomy (through the belly button), either with or without the removal of her cervix. Removal of the ovaries (and thus the loss of hormones) is not required to treat bleeding or pain resulting from fibroids.

Adenomyosis

Adenomyosis is endometriosis within the muscle wall of the uterus. The most common symptoms are painful periods with a very heavy flow, so heavy that anemia, or low blood count, can result. Adenomyosis is usually not a discrete lesion; more often, it is a diffuse network of branching endometrial glands, extending from the endometrium and invading the muscle wall of the uterus. These lesions have no real beginning or end. When you look at a cross-section of a uterus with adenomyosis, you can see varying concentrations of endometriosis within the muscle. An area with a high concentration of adenomyosis and little remaining normal muscle tissue is known as an adenomyoma.

A normal uterus is fairly hard and firm. A uterus with adenomyosis is usually slightly enlarged and soft or squishy to the touch, like a sponge. A careful medical history and physical exam might raise the possibility of adenomyosis. If the concentration and size of the adenomyosis is large enough, a sonogram (ultrasound) or MRI can be helpful in making the diagnosis; laparoscopic evaluation may also be helpful. When adenomyosis is present, the uterus often looks "sunburned" and blanches to the touch, just as when you press on sunburned skin. Examining the surgical specimen (after a hysterectomy, for instance) under a microscope is the only sure way of making an absolute diagnosis.

The treatment options are similar to those for endometriosis:

- *Observation* This means to just watch; do not start any treatment. It is an acceptable option if the symptoms are not severe.

- *Medical treatment* This includes birth control pills and GnRH agonists (found in medications such as Lupron and Synarel). The pills will lighten a woman's period and thus her symptoms. The GnRH agonists may temporarily alleviate the symptoms and even reduce the size of the adenomyosis. But the drug will not eliminate the adenomyosis, nor will it prevent continued growth if the GnRH is discontinued.

- *Conservative surgical treatment* It's possible to reconstruct the uterus during a myomectomy (surgery to remove fibroids), because fibroids are discrete lesions that can be completely removed. With an adenomyomectomy, however, reconstructing the uterus is usually not possible, because so much of the uterus has been destroyed. At best, this surgery will reduce the amount of adenomyosis. Due to the nature of the lesion, a significant amount of disease usually will remain, and it's likely that a patient who has this procedure will need to undergo additional surgery within a couple of years. A woman who is trying to get pregnant or is in the rare situation of having a single, well-defined adenomyoma, may be a candidate for this type of conservative surgical treatment. It may also be an acceptable option for a woman who is opposed to having a hysterectomy and does not mind undergoing repeated surgeries to maintain what is, in truth, a diseased organ.

- *Definitive surgical treatment with hysterectomy* This is the only option for truly curing a patient of adenomyosis. Having a hysterectomy is never a decision that should be taken lightly. Too many hysterectomies have been performed in the past. But others' wrongs should not prevent a patient from doing what is right for her. Severe symptoms will usually require the removal of the diseased organ—that is, a hysterectomy—both to obtain relief and to avoid the real possibility of repetitive surgeries. Because in most cases the ovaries are not removed, a hysterectomy for adenomyosis will not necessarily equal menopause.

Uterine Retroversion

Normally the uterus is tipped forward, toward the pubic bone. Uterine retroversion means that the uterus is tipped back. It is not always a problem; many patients with this condition have no symptoms. Some women experience pain with intercourse. That's because when the uterus is tipped back, the main part is positioned at the end of the vagina. The ovaries, which are attached to the top of the uterus, also are closer to the end of the vagina. Collisional dyspareunia is the medical term for the painful sex that occurs when the uterus gets hit with deep penetration. A uterine suspension with round ligament plication (shortening the ligament) will tip the uterus forward and out of the line of fire, so to speak, solving the problem for most women. This procedure is done with minimally invasive surgery through a laparoscope.

Pelvic Congestion

Pelvic congestion, uterine varicosities, and ovarian vein varicosities (varicose veins) are all variations of enlarged pelvic blood vessels. Varicose veins result in distension of the blood vessel, which is why you can see them in a leg. You know how distension of the bowel with gas can be painful; this distension can cause pain, too.

Vein varicosities in the ovaries can be treated without removal of or damage to any of the reproductive organs. When the veins of the uterus are involved, however, a hysterectomy may be required. One study showed a pain level with intercourse before surgery of 10/10 and a pain level after surgery of about 1/10.[48]

Abdominal-wall Neuropathy

The ilio-inguinal, ilio-hypogastric, and genital femoral nerves are found in the lower abdominal wall between the belly button and hipbone, down to the groin and upper leg. When these nerves are damaged, a nerve block or trigger-point injection can be helpful; often, a series of nerve blocks can ease the pain. In some cases, a technique called radiofrequency nerve ablation is used to provide longer-lasting relief. These are both office procedures.

Pudendal Neuropathy and Pudendal Nerve Entrapment (PNE)

The pudendal nerve is located along the side of the vagina. This nerve has three basic branches: an anterior branch, to the clitoris; a middle branch, to the vaginal and vulvar area; and a posterior branch, to the

---

48   Beard RW, Kennedy RG, Gangar KF, Stones RW, Rogers V, Reginald PW, Anderson M. Bilateral oophorectomy and hysterectomy in the treatment of intractable pelvic pain associated with pelvic congestion. *British Journal of Obstetrics and Gynecology*. 1991;98(10):988-992.

anus. Pain can be present in any portion of the nerve if it becomes damaged or entrapped. The pain is often worse when the patient is sitting.

A diagnosis of pudendal neuropathy can be made if a pudendal nerve block relieves the pain. Often, a doctor will prescribe a combination of pudendal nerve blocks and pelvic-floor physical therapy; in some cases, I have found radiofrequency ablation of the pudendal nerve to be helpful (explained on page 135). While a couple of medical centers offer pudendal nerve entrapment surgery to provide relief, this surgery is considered rather radical and of questionable efficacy.

Food Allergies and Food Sensitivities

While technically different, food allergies and food sensitivities can result in similar types of problems. A food allergy, such as to seafood, is mediated by the immune system: the patient may break out in a rash and/or may experience difficulty breathing. A food sensitivity, such as lactose intolerance, has an end-organ response: the patient reacts to the food with, for example, a spasm of the bowel.

Gluten is a protein found in wheat, rye, barley, oat bran, and wheat germ. While it can cause celiac disease, gluten is also a leading cause of food sensitivity. The symptoms are very similar. With celiac disease, the lining of the gastrointestinal tract becomes damaged, but the pain with gluten sensitivity—such as severe bowel pain, up to a level of 10/10—can be just as severe. Other symptoms include bloating, diarrhea, skin problems, headaches, even neurologic symptoms, such as irritation and anxiety. Food sensitivities can also contribute to or cause pain in the vulvar area and make interstitial cystitis symptoms worse.

Blood tests can be used to diagnose celiac disease. Food allergies can be diagnosed with blood tests and some skin tests. Food sensitivities can be diagnosed with a particular type of allergy skin test known as provocation and neutralization testing. The best way to diagnose food sensitivity is to eliminate the food in question for two weeks and then eat a lot of it. If the symptoms get better, only to return when you start eating that food again, it's likely a food sensitivity.

Ovarian Remnant

This term refers to a painful condition that occurs when the ovary is surgically removed but part of it remains in place. This happens more often than you might think, especially when the ovary is surrounded by scar tissue. The ovary itself looks similar to scar tissue, so it can be very difficult to tell which is which. And the ovaries are quite close to the major blood vessel going into each leg, which may result in the surgeon not getting close enough to the blood vessel to remove all of the ovary because of concern about cutting a hole in this large blood vessel. Dissection of all scar tissue away from the blood vessel helps reduce the chance of an ovarian remnant

Sometimes the ovarian remnant can be diagnosed with a sonogram (ultrasound) or by persistently elevated estrogen levels, as determined by a blood test. Surgical removal of the ovary and surrounding scar tissue usually relieves the pain.

Foreign Body

I have found several cases of pelvic pain caused by foreign material left in the body after surgery—most often, on purpose. Two of the most common examples are surgical staples and mesh.

Quick and efficient, surgical staples are used by many if not most surgeons. Most surgeons performing laparoscopic hysterectomies and appendectomies, for instance, use surgical staples. One use of larger staples is to clamp a blood vessel to stop bleeding. This is not usually a problem, but if the staple is close to something like the ureter (the urine tube from the kidney to the bladder), the patient can feel pain as the ureter peristalses, or moves, which it does on a regular basis.

Early in my career, I had a patient who had been to many doctors without getting rid of her pelvic pain. We were getting ready to do a patient-assisted laparoscopy to map the pain; I was meeting with her before the procedure to answer questions. As we looked at an X-ray from one of her previous surgeries, she asked about the staples in her pelvis. Could they be the reason for her pain? I reassured her that staples would not have caused a problem. Boy, was I wrong! One staple was right on her ureter, and every time I flicked it during the

PAL, it re-created the pain she felt whenever her ureter moved. I removed the staple, and her pain was gone.

Surgical staples are made primarily of titanium, but some contain a little bit of nickel as well. It is uncommon but known in dentistry for some patients to feel pain from implants with nickel. I believe the same thing can happen with surgical staples. While this may not yet be a proven fact, I always remove any surgical staples I find. And I never use them during GYN surgery, because of the risk of postoperative pain.

Mesh looks something like the screen you put on a window. It's used primarily for fixing hernias, which are little holes in the body, although hernia repairs, especially small ones, don't always require the use of mesh. I have found that women with pelvic pain who have inguinal, or groin, hernias repaired with mesh are at risk of developing a new pain as a result of the mesh scarring into surrounding nerves.

Mesh is used in other areas of the body as well. I had one patient who experienced recurrent bowel obstruction, with nausea and vomiting, with her period. When we did her surgery, I found that in an earlier surgery, to repair a belly button hernia, mesh had been left hanging down into her abdomen, where her bowel scarred to the mesh. Using a CO_2 laser, I gently removed the bowel from the mesh without damaging the bowel. I cut off the extra mesh and, yes, her pain and symptoms of bowel obstruction resolved. This is just one more example of why, with pelvic pain, it is so important to listen to the patient, keep an open mind, and use all appropriate methods to treat her.

Hernias

Groin hernias include inguinal, obturator, and femoral hernias. The inguinal is the most common, although in my experience, it is a fairly uncommon cause of pelvic pain. This condition has been overdiagnosed, with much unnecessary pain from mesh placement. If such hernias are present, they should be treated without mesh.

It is also possible to get painful hernias in the abdominal wall. These can include incisional hernias, belly button hernias, and ventral hernias, a condition where the "six-pack" muscles separate in the middle, which can happen after pregnancy.

Appendicitis

Most cases of appendicitis are acute, meaning they come on quickly— usually over a period of hours—sending the patient to the emergency room, where the appendix is removed in emergency surgery. Obviously, these cases are rarely confused with chronic pelvic pain and endometriosis. But sometimes the opposite can occur: a patient is thought to have endometriosis pain and is sent home, only to have her appendix rupture, which is serious.

I have had a couple of cases of what appeared to be a low-grade, chronic infection in the appendix. In these cases, the patient had pain in the area of the appendix—the right side of the pelvic area, between the belly button and the hip bone—and we reproduced that pain with palpation at PAL. Once the appendix was removed, the pain was better, and the pathology report showed signs of chronic infection. Pathology reports have also shown microscopic endo in the appendix. For these reasons—including appendicitis being mistaken for endo—when a significant part of the patient's pain is in the area of the appendix, I recommend it be removed.

Gastrointestinal Problems: Motility Problems, Redundant Colon, Diverticulitis, Anal Fissure

Bowel problems are common in patients with pelvic pain. Food allergies and sensitivities, which I discussed earlier, can result in significant bowel problems. Bowel motility refers to how the bowel moves; a bowel can become spastic, for instance, and that will cause pain. A partial bowel obstruction resulting from adhesions can be quite painful—even if all the different X-rays and tests come back "normal," which can happen unless the obstruction is pretty bad. Rarely, redundant colon—that is, an extra length of colon—can become a problem, leading to severe constipation and pain. Diverticulitis, when a small pouch forms in the colon and becomes infected, can be painful. An anal fissure is a crack in the lining of the anus, often as a result of constipation, which can cause severe pain with bowel movements.

Lyme Disease

Lyme is a well-documented infectious disease resulting from tick bites. Chronic Lyme disease, though, is a controversial area, with two camps of doctors who oppose each other in their thinking. On one side is a group of "Lyme literate" doctors who diagnose and treat chronic Lyme disease. Most of these doctors belong to ILADS, the International Lyme and Associated Disease Society. On the other side are most infectious-disease doctors and members of IDSA, the Infectious Diseases Society of America, who feel that Lyme disease does not exist in a chronic form. In my opinion, the truth is probably somewhere in between. I have had patients affected by Lyme disease and know that treatment from Lyme doctors has helped them.

As you may have guessed, the symptoms of Lyme and endometriosis have quite a bit of overlap. Without going into detail, standard testing for Lyme disease is complex and controversial—including the fact that the recommended approach doesn't conform to the standard criteria for medical testing—and frequently, standard tests will be falsely negative. I advise patients to become educated on as many aspects of this disease and its various treatments as they can.

Generalized Visceral Hypersensitivity

The word *viscera* refers to the internal organs. *Hypersensitivity* means abnormally sensitive, such as when you get a bad sunburn and pressure that wouldn't normally hurt or even be felt is painful. With generalized visceral hypersensitivity, the entire inside of the body hurts. This is usually because inappropriate signals are being sent by the nervous system, creating types of neuropathic pain or centralized pain. (See chapter seven.)

With some patients who I diagnosed using PAL, everything hurt; we could not re-create the pain in one specific area. Since we couldn't locate a specific anatomic problem, further surgery was not in the patient's best interest. In those cases, it is better to try using mind-body medicine, medications, physical therapy, and pain management, possibly including interventional pain management, with pain pumps or nerve stimulators.

Vulvodynia

The vulva is the area surrounding the outside of the vagina. *Vulvodynia* means "pain of the vulva." There are two general types of vulvodynia. Patients with generalized vulvodynia can experience pain anywhere on the vulva between the thighs. It can involve the entire area or specific, isolated areas. The pain can be intermittent or constant. Vulvar vestibulitis involves pain of the vestibule, the small area around the opening of the vagina inside the labia minora, or inner lips. Pain is present only with pressure on the area, such as with intercourse or tampon insertion.

In most cases, the precise cause of vulvodynia is not known. A variety of common chemicals, including those found in laundry soap, fabric softener, perfumes, and dyes, can cause pain of the vulva. Some foods can cause pain and irritation; again, elimination and reintroduction of foods can determine if a particular food is a contributing factor. Several treatments are available, but there is no known cure. A good pelvic-floor physical therapist can be very helpful in treating vulvodynia. More information is available through the National Vulvodynia Association.

One thing I have learned from experience is to listen to and trust the patient, keep an open mind, and use all diagnostic and therapeutic tools available, as appropriate for each situation.

✿ ✿ ✿

"Meeting my doctor put me at ease. I was never dismissed, and he believed what I told him. During my first appointment, my examination was completely different. He was trying to reproduce the pain in order to identify its origin. Through the process, I was treated with respect." —Lillyth

"When I met my doctor, he took his time. I felt understood, and I was relieved that I was being heard. I came back and had a PAP and an ultrasound. The doctor saw a cyst immediately and knew I had endometriosis. The endo had eaten through my vaginal wall. Why hadn't the other doc-tors noticed that?" —I-Li

"My doctor did an exam called pain mapping. There were places he touched me that brought me right off the table! But he was able to pinpoint where I had endometriosis right away." —Kelli

CHAPTER SIX

Getting the Best Treatment for Endometriosis

As we've seen, the best treatment for endometriosis involves the whole patient, and a good endometriosis specialist will have a team of professionals either on hand or available by referral to support the patient. The idea is not to just rid her of disease, but also to restore her to all-around good health. Depending on her needs, I might refer a patient to a pain-management specialist, nutritionist, physical therapist, psychologist or counselor, gastroenterologist, urologist, or complementary-medicine practitioner. It's all about the big picture of her health.

But in this chapter, I'm going to focus on the medical and surgical treatment of endometriosis. You can't restore a patient to good health until you rid her of the disease.

Medications for Treating Endometriosis

The only way to get rid of endometriosis is to remove it with laparoscopic surgery with wide excision. But that isn't always the first treatment I'll turn to. As always, it depends on the individual and the degree of her symptoms. If I see a patient who says, "You know, I feel pretty good; it's just that my periods have been getting a little worse, and they're starting to slow me down a bit," I'm not going to suggest surgery right away. I will usually try hormonal treatments to see if we can calm the endo down, at least for a time.

Birth Control Pills

For a patient whose symptoms are not severe, I often prescribe birth control pills first, because the side effects, if any, are usually mild, and the cost is so low that while the pill may not be a permanent fix, it's a reasonable approach for the time being.

Birth control pills help control the disease because they reduce the amount of estrogen in the system, and estrogen feeds endometriosis. In healthy women, estrogen is what builds up the lining in the uterus; progesterone stabilizes the lining. If you take an oral contraceptive pill every day, you're turning the ovaries off. Even though the pill contains hormones, your body is exposed to about half as many hormones as normal. Oral contraceptives have been shown to provide some pain relief in about 75 to 89 percent of the patients studied.[49] But they do nothing to reduce or remove the endometriosis.

Of course, the Pill has well-known side effects, and some women cannot tolerate oral contraceptives. If you are one of these women, you are not alone. I estimate that 10 to 20 percent of the patients I see with endometriosis and pelvic pain have such severe side effects from the Pill that they can't take it. These side effects include nausea, vomiting, bleeding, irritability, high blood pressure, headache, dysphoria (feeling emotionally down; the opposite of euphoria), and, over time, decreased or nonexistent sex drive. These are not trivial symptoms.

With a patient who can tolerate the Pill, I almost always start out—at least for the first month or two—by having her take it cyclically. Each month, she takes 21 days of hormonal pills and seven days of sugar pills, getting her period while she's taking the sugar pills. I start with this approach to minimize unwanted-bleeding problems. Since a woman on the Pill gets only half the normal amount of estrogen each month, her endometrium (uterine lining) becomes about half as thick. This transition to a thinner lining is why some women experience breakthrough bleeding the first month or two they are on the Pill; it is the most common side effect at that stage.

---

49 Olive DL. Medical treatment: alternatives to Danazol. In: Schenken RS, ed. *Endometriosis: Contemporary Concepts in Clinical Management*. Philadelphia PA: JB Lippincott; 1989:189-211.

Once a patient has a couple of regular periods, I have her take the Pill continuously, meaning she skips the sugar pills and takes a hormone pill every day, without a break. I tell patients to continue taking the hormone pills until they begin spotting or cramping or start a period. When this happens, they stop the Pill for five days and then start taking it again. Some women can go indefinitely without a period; others seem to have a period every four weeks no matter what. It is okay to go without a period, because the hormones—the estrogen and progesterone—are in balance. No toxins are building up, nor is the reproductive system being damaged. It will all work the same when you're ready to get pregnant. For patients who feel well other than having painful periods, this approach can be quite effective.

I also frequently prescribe the Pill after endometriosis surgery. While we do not completely understand what causes endometriosis, if some of it does come from retrograde menstruation, taking the Pill will help to decrease the amount of bleeding back up inside the body. The body's scavenger cells, the macrophage, seem to be underactive or lazy in endometriosis patients. If their job is smaller—if there are fewer endometrial cells to clean up, because there is less bleeding—then perhaps there's a better chance the macrophage will get all the endo cells and not leave any behind to turn into endometriosis.

Lupron

In its most recent Management of Endometriosis Practice Bulletin, the American College of Obstetrics and Gynecology (ACOG) allows the use of Lupron, if birth control pills are not helpful, before a laparoscopy is performed to diagnose and treat endometriosis. Many physicians, including myself, disagree with this practice. Indeed, a fair amount of controversy surrounds treatment of endometriosis and the use of this drug. Even with the risk of severe side effects, many physicians routinely prescribe it without first diagnosing and removing the endo, which in the majority of cases will quickly solve the problem.

Lupron is the brand name of a drug in a class of drugs called gonadotropin-releasing hormone (GnRH) agonists. It is given in a shot every month or once every three months, depending on the dose. It acts by altering the brain chemistry in such a way that the ovaries temporarily stop working, thereby preventing ovulation and hormone production, and the woman goes into a medical menopause. This is not like the gradual change of natural menopause. With Lupron, bam—just like that, the woman goes into menopause, with all of its symptoms. Hot flashes, fatigue, depression, mood swings, vaginal dryness, headaches, insomnia, and decreased sex drive are common on this drug. Less common are acne, dizziness, diarrhea, painful joints, short-term memory loss, and nausea.[50] Many feel add-back therapy—low-dose estrogen and/or progesterone replacement—alleviates these symptoms.

Many patients have told me the side effects were worse than the pain the Lupron was supposed to treat. The long-term effects include bone-density loss, which is why US and Canadian regulatory agencies have a six month limit on the use of drugs like Lupron.

Lupron does not cure endometriosis; if it did, it might be worth going through the six months of hell. At best, it temporarily suppresses endometriosis. Some patients get pain relief, especially if the pain is primarily with their periods. But once the ovaries start working again, the endometriosis reactivates, and the pain usually returns. Twenty years ago, doctors believed that if the pain didn't go away on Lupron, the problem wasn't endometriosis. During the 1990s I operated on many women who had persistent pain while they were taking Lupron. I found active endometriosis in virtually every one, as documented by the pathologist who looked at the endometrial implants under a microscope. At the time, I did not know why this was the case. In 1996 the first study came out reporting that endometriosis can produce its own estrogen; it can promote its own growth.[51] This research explained our findings! Lupron can't touch the estrogen the endometriosis creates.

In many ways Lupron is very controversial with wide-ranging opinions about it. One could write a book solely on Lupron and all of the issues related to its use; it has advantages and disadvantages. Many

---

50 Adamson GD, Pasta DJ. Surgical treatment of endometriosis-associated infertility: meta-analysis compared with survival analysis. *American Journal of Obstetrics and Gynecology*. 1994;171(6):1488-1505.

51 Noble LS, Simpson ER, Johns A, Bulun SE. Aromatase expression in endometriosis. *Journal of Clinical Endocrinology and Metabolism*. 1996;81(1):174-179.

people, including physicians have many misconceptions regarding this drug. As with any other treatment option, it is important to understand potential benefits, risks, and how they apply to any individual situation. Personally I am not a fan of this medication, as it seems to me the benefits rarely outweigh the potential negatives, especially when compared to other treatment options. Some physicians for whom I have great respect and are very good endometriosis doctors feel that Lupron, when used properly, can provide good benefit to certain select endometriosis patients.

It seems that many of the problems surrounding the use of Lupron stem out of misunderstanding endometriosis in general and the role of Lupron in particular. All too often, general OB/GYNs see Lupron as providing better results with less down side than what is actually the case. Too often Lupron is provided as the only treatment alternative. Unfortunately, and not uncommonly, it is also used inappropriately to confirm a diagnosis of endometriosis or to determine if the patient really has another primary cause of her pain, including a psychological one. This is one important reason that, in my opinion, endometriosis should be a sub-specialty—one that provides a level of expertise in providing care to patients with endometriosis that exceeds the current situation with general OB/GYNs who do not have the same level of expertise and knowledge.

For example, I was reviewing a new patient's medical records recently and came across a physician who reported doing a laparoscopy where he saw endo, but he "could not get it all out safely." When the woman's pain persisted, he prescribed Lupron. When her pain continued, the doctor told her it must be a bowel problem. When she insisted it was endometriosis pain, the doctor told her that while she was on Lupron, it was impossible to have pain related to endometriosis. The patient's husband now believes she is just trying to avoid having sex with him.

Is this really the best we can do for endo patients? Why does the American College of Obstetrics and Gynecology recommend using Lupron?

While not cheap (about $675 for a one-month shot and $2075 for a 3-month shot), Lupron is less expensive than surgery. It also seems to provide comparable results to the less-than-optimal quality of surgery (and thus relatively poor results) of the average endometriosis surgery.[52] In response to current laparoscopic surgical skills of OB/GYNs, a respected GYN scientific journal concluded, "Residency programs in the United States continue to provide inadequate training ..." The uncomfortable truth seems to be that many if not most general OB/GYN doctors are using either outdated surgical techniques or do not have sufficient surgical skills to completely remove the endometriosis. With disease still left in the body, the symptoms either persist or quickly return.

Fortunately, there is a third alternative to mediocre medical or surgical treatment not mentioned by the ACOG bulletin, which is to refer patients with this challenging, complex disease to a doctor who specializes in the treatment of endometriosis (a sub-specialist).

❁ ❁ ❁

"I had surgery for an ovarian cyst. The surgeon told me I also had Stage IV endometriosis, the worst, and said that I would 'never get it all out of there.' The treatment was Lupron. As a good patient, I took the Lupron shot and descended into a new kind of hell: immediate chemical menopause, crying, panic attacks, severe insomnia, hot flashes, depression, and thoughts of suicide. I placed a phone call to the doctor. I was told by the nurse that there was nothing else they could do for me." —Elizabeth

---

52   Pain and Quality of Life Survey, commissioned by the UK Endometriosis All-Party Parliamentary Group and presented at the Ninth World Congress on Endometriosis, Maastricht, The Netherlands, 2005.

Danazol

This drug is derived from testosterone, the male hormone, and sold under the trade names Danocrine and Cyclomen. The way the drug seems to work is by suppressing the normal signals from the pituitary gland to the ovary, decreasing estrogen and also inhibiting the enzymes responsible for producing estrogen in the ovaries and adrenal glands. Danazol seems to have an influence on the immune system as well, decreasing the inflammatory response to pelvic endometriosis.

Danazol was approved by the FDA to treat endometriosis and has been used since the 1970s. Danazol gets absorbed rapidly by the gastrointestinal tract, so it has to be taken two or three times a day. I generally prescribe it to women who are not in a position to go through surgery, or for whom the Pill hasn't worked and their periods are the primary problem. The advantage of danazol is that because it's short acting, if it's not a good fit for you, it's out of your system fast. But it can have side effects, such as oily skin, acne, hair growth, and headaches. It can also decrease good cholesterol (HDL) and have negative effects on liver function and carbohydrate metabolism. Danazol is not natural, and while it is not a great treatment, sometimes it is the best choice given the other options.

Progesterone Drugs

The idea behind the class of drugs called progestogens is that they counteract the effect of estrogen on the endometrial tissue. Depo-Provera (sometimes known as the birth control shot) is a long-acting form of progesterone. The most common side effects of Depo-Provera are breakthrough bleeding, weight gain, and depression. If you get uncomfortable side effects from the drug, you have to live with them for months. Some doctors use it to treat endometriosis, though I haven't found that it relieves the pain much.

I have found that some patients do well on bio-identical progesterone, taken orally or via topical cream on a daily basis, if their symptoms fluctuate with their hormonal levels during the month and they can't tolerate the birth control pill. If side effects are encountered, the medicine can be stopped and out of the patient's body within a couple of days.

Aromatase Enzyme Inhibitors

These drugs, including letrozole and anastrozole, are used in treating breast cancer and ovarian cancer in postmenopausal women. Because the aromatase enzyme inhibitor blocks all estrogen, including the estrogen the endo is producing, these drugs are sometimes prescribed for endometriosis. They have the same side effects that Lupron does. I do have a couple of patients I have treated with aromatase enzyme inhibitors, though. Every patient's situation is different, and some cases are highly complex. This is another treatment for the right situation.

Laparoscopic Surgery

The pervasive misunderstanding as to what constitutes good endometriosis surgery is a huge part of why so many women with endo continue to live lives of pain and suffering. I will try to shed light on the subject in a way that both physicians and patients can understand.

Endometriosis is not a cancer, but it is a collection of benign tumors. As with all tumors, they remain in the body until they are removed. The only scientifically proven method of removing endometriosis is surgery; if the surgery is done correctly, it is possible to remove all the endometriosis. The problem is, too often the surgery is done incorrectly.

Gynecologic cancer surgery is so different from routine gynecologic surgery that there is a subspecialty training and certification process for these surgeons. Endometriosis surgery—which has more in common with cancer surgery than most other types of surgery and is just as complex—is very different from the kinds of surgeries most gynecologists are trained to perform. It warrants its own subspecialty training and certification. Unfortunately, treating endometriosis and pelvic pain is not a recognized specialty.

Historically, infertility specialists called reproductive endocrinologists treated endometriosis patients. They were known for their advanced (compared to general OB/GYNs) laparoscopic skills. But over the years, fertility treatment has moved away from surgery and toward in vitro fertilization. Today endometriosis is treated less often by reproductive endocrinologists and more often by general OB/GYNs—which means that unspecialized, general OB/GYN doctors are performing what can be very specialized, difficult surgery. I think the current medical/ insurance system is unfairly expecting them to treat this disease; it isn't right to expect these specialized skills of general doctors. I say this with the utmost respect for general OB/GYNs. Most are good people and good doctors. As discussed at the end of chapter four, it is becoming very clear from recent scientific data that the surgical training doctors receive in residency for even basic laparoscopic procedures is woefully inadequate. Some general OB/GYNs have obtained the surgical skills to treat the disease well, but they're the exceptions.

Wide Excision

The most important concept in treating endometriosis effectively is completely removing the disease from the body, which is usually done with wide excision at surgery. Excision means that the lesion is excised or cut out. Wide excision means that a margin of normal-appearing tissue is removed along with the lesion, to ensure that any microscopic disease that extends out from the visible lesion is also eliminated.

Many studies have shown the presence of endometriosis in normal tissue surrounding visible endometriosis.[53, 54, 55, 56] We all know that if what we thought was a simple mole was actually a melanoma (skin cancer), the doctor removing it would cut out not only the pigmented area, he or she would remove a zone of normal-appearing tissue with the melanoma, because of the very good chance that it contained a few cancer cells. This is the best approach for removing all the cancer.

The same thing is true with endometriosis. A zone of normal tissue should be removed through a wide excision. In my experience, about two-thirds of normal-looking specimens next to visible endometriosis

---

53   Murphy AA, Guizick DS, Rock JA. Microscopic peritoneal endometriosis. *Fertility and Sterility*. 1989;51(6):1072-1074.

54   Murphy AA, Green WR, Bobbie D, dela Cruz ZC, Rock JA. Unsuspected endometriosis documented by scanning electron microscopy in visually normal peritoneum. *Fertility and Sterility*. 1986;46(3):522-524.

55   Brosens IA, Vasquez G, Grodts S, Scanning electron microscopy study of the pelvic peritoneum in unexplained infertility and endometriosis. *Fertility and Sterility*. 1984;41:21S Abstract 48.

56   Vasques G, Cornillie F, Brosens IA. Peritoneal endometriosis: scanning electron microscopy and histology of minimal pelvic endometriotic lesions. *Fertility and Sterility*. 1984;42(5):696-703.

show microscopic endo when examined by a pathologist. This means that even if all visible endometriosis is removed, but without wide excision, two-thirds of these patients will have microscopic endometriosis remaining after surgery. When the disease stays in the body, even in such small quantities, those cells continue to grow, and the symptoms either persist or come back fairly quickly.

Removing only some of the endometriosis is just like pulling the tops off weeds and leaving the roots behind. Your garden will be full of weeds again in no time. But if you use the best techniques and carefully pull all the weeds out by the roots, your garden will be free of weeds. The risk of new weeds coming in and taking hold can be minimized or eliminated by taking steps to optimize the health of your garden. In the same way, good health practices can minimize the chance of recurring endometriosis.

Figure 2 describes conceptually the critical issue of complete versus partial removal of disease. Say the disease took more than 9 years to reach a certain stage. In this example, when only half is removed, the disease will grow back to the pre-operative state in only 8 months (0.7 years)! If 90 percent of the endometriosis is removed, we have gained only 2.3 years. This figure also explains why a patient's symptoms can come back so quickly with incomplete removal of the endometriosis. It has to do with the concepts of cell growth and cell number.

Figure 2. Example of Exponential Curve of Cell Growth

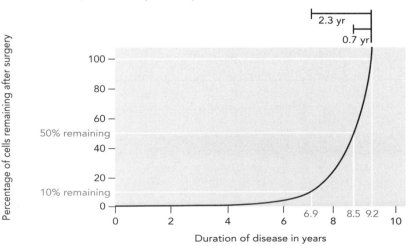

When cells grow and divide, they do so at a constant rate. Each cell type has a specific doubling time, which is the amount of time it takes to grow and divide from one cell into two. Those two cells will divide and multipy exponentially, becoming 4 cells, then 8, then 16, 32, 64, and so on. In 10 divisions, the cell number will go from one to more than a thousand. In another 19 divisions, the cell number will be more than one million. After another 10 divisions, there will be more than one billion cells.

Cell growth follows this exponential curve, changing slowly at first, changing rapidly after a critical cell mass is reached. Removing only half the disease means there is still a critical mass. Cell regrowth to pre-surgical levels can occur in a matter of months. No wonder the most common surgical treatment for endometriosis—coagulation, which removes just part of the diseased tissue—has such poor results and such a high "recurrence" rate.

It's important to make a distinction between the likelihood of a true recurrence after a good surgery, which is very low (perhaps 15 to 20 percent over five years), and of endometriosis continuing to grow after incomplete treatment. The patients who have a rapid "recurrence" are almost always those whose physicians didn't get all the endo out in the first place.

The idea behind successful surgical treatment is so simple: get all the endometriosis out of the body. So why is it so difficult to achieve this result? Consider the following checklist of potential problem areas, any one of which, alone or in combination with others, can cause less than optimal surgical results.

- *Diagnosis* Mild forms of endometriosis, including Stage I and Stage II endo, can be so subtle they are simply overlooked. Surprisingly, advanced types of invasive endometriosis can also be missed; they can invade the body in out-of-sight places and some types can be surrounded by vital structures not easy to separate from the endo.

- *Surgical technique* Even with Stage I or Stage II endo, wide areas of the pelvis can be covered with small implants. (Think of a cup of sand dropped on the floor. The grains will spread everywhere.) Wide excision needs to be performed in these cases, although surgeons are often reluctant to do so. Wide excision with large margins should be used when removing "microscopic" endometriosis; coagulation techniques are not well suited to this, as I will explain below. Advanced Stage III and Stage IV invasive endometriosis should be treated only by endo specialists with the advanced surgical skills needed for this type of surgery.

- *Surgical assistance* With many cases of endometriosis, especially advanced cases, it takes three hands to do a good job. An assistant trained in advanced laparoscopic techniques will help gain the necessary exposure (view) and provide an additional pair of hands.

- *Pathology skill* After the surgery, in a process that takes a couple of days, a pathologist provides the surgeon with a report detailing what was found in the tissue the surgeon removed. The pathologist tells the surgeon whether the tissue does, in fact, contain endometriosis. The pathologist's assessment isn't always correct, however; that depends on how well he or she handles and processes the tissue to prepare it for viewing under the microscope. In my experience, many pathologists are not as careful or detail oriented as we would like. If the pathologist does not see the endometriosis that really is in the tissue, he or she can mistakenly tell the surgeon there was no endo. Over time, given enough such false negative reports, the endo surgeon may come to doubt his or her own perceptions in surgery and fail to remove endo that's actually there.

Effective Surgery

To reiterate, endometriosis isn't necessarily a few obvious lesions. Endo can hide in the corners of the pelvis, where it's hard to get to. There can be lots of little endometrial implants scattered about. In the worst cases, the entire pelvis is full of scar tissue and adhesions, and organs are stuck together.

So what makes a surgery effective? First of all, the skill and experience of the surgeon. It takes years of doing advanced laparoscopic surgery to be able to fully identify and remove all the endometriosis, to sweep the house clean. It takes highly specialized techniques to perform successful surgery on a woman with advanced endo; this can take an hour or two or, in the worst cases, as long as 10 hours. It can be like erasing freckles from a redhead. It calls for patience.

Some OB/GYNs, especially when faced with advanced forms of endometriosis, open the patient up. They do a "bikini incision," a laparotomy—the big cut. You might find it surprising that with this kind of surgery, the surgeon cannot see nearly as well as during a laparoscopy. When I look into a woman's pelvis using the laparoscope, it magnifies up to eight times and displays the image on a large, high-definition, wide-screen monitor.

I work with an anesthesiologist, an assistant surgeon, a laser technician, an operating-room nurse, and a couple of operating-room technicians, who get any supplies we need. Before surgery, my team talks the patient through each step until she is asleep. Laparoscopic surgery is done under general anesthesia, so everything I'm describing from here on is what happens once the patient is asleep. (I give my patients a video of their surgery, so they can see it for themselves.)

After the patient goes under the anesthesia, a breathing tube is put in through her mouth, and the anesthesia machine breaths for her. I typically make three small incisions (one in the belly button and one a little in from each hip bone where it is hidden under a bikini), for the laparoscope and the associated instruments. Once we turn the laparoscope on, we have that great view of the pelvis on two big video screens. We have the latest, most advanced video system in my operating room. The quality and clarity of the picture is really quite amazing.

First we do a systematic evaluation of the abdominal and pelvic cavities. This involves exploring all the folds and nooks and crannies inside the pelvis. Many people think that finding endometriosis in the pelvis is similar to opening a door and looking into the room to see if any pictures are on the wall (pictures representing endometriosis in this example). The pelvis is actually more like your bed before it is made in the morning. Looking to see if there is a quarter in the sheets and covers is a better example of finding endometriosis in the pelvis.

Usually you would have to pull the sheets straight up and look in between the layers to find the quarter. I carefully inspect the peritoneum (the Saran Wrap-like lining inside the body) one area at a time, so that no area is missed. With endo, very small, hard-to-see lesions can cause excruciating pain. A surgeon must be very thorough and meticulous to find it all.

The lesions can be dark, pigmented spots, similar to a blood blister, or orange, black, white, red, or clear, like tiny water balloons. The disease can look like specks of salt or leathery scar tissue. With sufficient time and the proper magnification, it can all be found. Any scar tissue must be found and removed as well.

Removing the Endometriosis

Now we're getting to the most complicated part: the technical details. Stick with me—once you understand the best way to remove endometriosis during surgery, you'll be much better equipped to advocate for the approach you want your doctor to take. See Figure 3 below which illustrates the basic concepts of endometriosis surgery and surgical techniques.

Figure 3. Basic Concepts of Endometriosis Surgery and Surgical Techniques

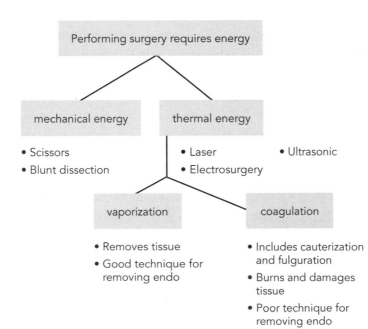

Energy and Its Effects on Tissue

Trimming paper with scissors is an example of mechanical energy. The heat and steam of an iron taking the wrinkles out of a dress is an example of thermal energy. In surgery, mechanical energy comes from the muscles of the surgeon, separating, pulling apart, or cutting tissue. Thermal energy can come from several different devices, including lasers, surgical electricity (electrosurgery), and the harmonic scalpel, which uses high-intensity sound waves.

When tissue is exposed to thermal energy, one of two things can happen—vaporization or coagulation—depending on the intensity (strength) of the heat and how fast it is transmitted. Vaporization is the process by which solids and liquids inside the treated cells are turned into a gaseous form (vapor). It occurs with a rapid rise in temperature—in the tissue, to above 100 degrees centigrade. If you leave an empty pan on a hot burner until the pan is extremely hot and then dump a small amount of water in, swoosh, the water will instantly turn into steam; there won't be any water left in the pan. A surgical laser, delivering a very concentrated packet of light energy, instantaneously boils the water in the cell (cells are mostly water, with some proteins and other substances). The water turns into steam, which expands in volume by more than a thousandfold, causing the cell to burst and disappear into a fog-like mixture of water vapor and suspended cellular proteins.

Vaporization can be used to remove endometriosis through two different surgical techniques: Thermal Excision by Linear Vaporization (TEL-V), the official complete descriptive term, or more simply, Excisional Vaporization (EV); and Ablative—or Area—Vaporization (AV) as shown in Figures 4 and 5 on the next page.

Figure 4. Thermal Excision by
Linear Vaporization (TEL-V or EV)

Figure 5. Ablative Vaporization (AV)

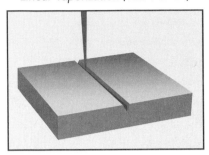

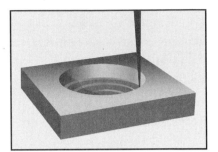

Thermal Excision by Linear Vaporization (TEL-V or EV) acts as a light knife, cutting as you might with scissors, removing (vaporizing) a line of cells in the process. If you cut between the endometriosis and the normal tissue, you can remove the endometriosis from the body. Ablative Vaporization (AV) acts like an eraser, causing all of the endometriosis to be removed by vaporization of all the cells.

The effect on the tissue remaining after the disease is removed, whether by EV or AV, is the same. Excisional Vaporization (EV) and Ablative Vaporization (AV) are equally good techniques for removing endo, so long as no cells are missed and all the cells are vaporized when using AV.

The following diagrams should help explain these concepts. Figure 6 illustrates a cross-section of tissue. The dark gray represents the endometriosis, including microscopic dots. The medium gray represents the surrounding margin of normal-looking tissue, which must be removed to make sure no microscopic endo remains. The black line represents the thin line of tissue vaporized next to the normal tissue (light gray) that's left behind after the endo is removed. (The white area at the top simply represents air inside the body.)

Let's use an example of balloons to better understand the concepts of EV and AV. Say we have a room full of balloons that are stuck together. The left side of the room is filled with red balloons; the right side, with blue balloons; there's a line of yellow balloons down the middle. The red balloons represent endometriosis, and the blue balloons represent normal tissue. If we pop all the yellow balloons and remove all the red balloons (remember, they are stuck together, as one unit), this is like Excisional Vaporization (EV). If we start at the edge of the room and work our way to the middle, popping all the red balloons and then all the yellow balloons (the last row of balloons we pop), this is like Ablative Vaporization (AV). In both cases, all that remains is the blue balloons.

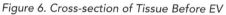

Figure 6. Cross-section of Tissue Before EV

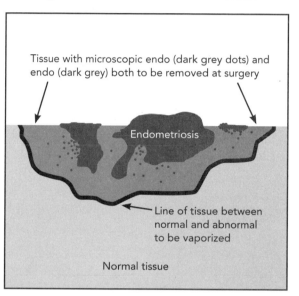

Figure 7 shows a line of tissue vaporized. This is the first step in EV. At this point, the endometriosis and surrounding margin of tissue are detached from the normal tissue.

Figure 7. Vaporized Line of Tissue (first step in EV)

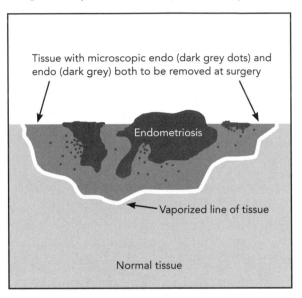

Figure 8 shows the endometriosis and surrounding tissue being removed.

Figure 8. Removal of Tissue Excised by EV

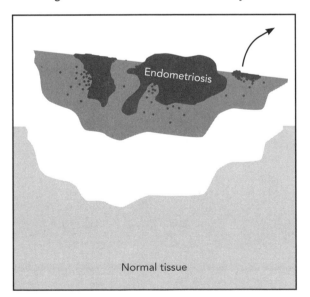

Finally, in Figure 9, we can see that only normal tissue remains. The appearance of the remaining normal tissue is the same whether the endometriosis was removed by EV or AV (see figures 9 and 14).

Figure 9. Normal Tissue Left After Excision with EV

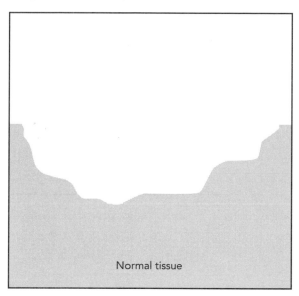

Figures 10 through 14 represent the process using Ablative—or Area—Vaporization. With AV, vaporization starts at the surface and works down, cell layer by cell layer, to the same line of tissue that would be vaporized using EV. With EV, the piece of tissue disappears. With AV, it goes up in a cloud of steam.

Figure 10. Cross-section of Tissue Before AV

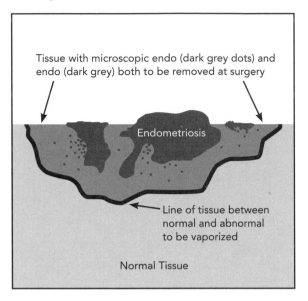

Figure 11. Beginning to Ablate Tissue by AV

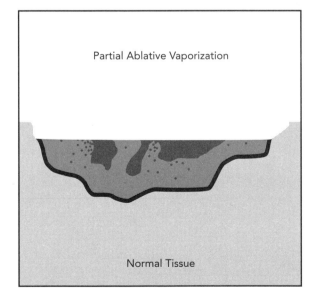

Figure 12. Further Ablation of the Lesion by AV

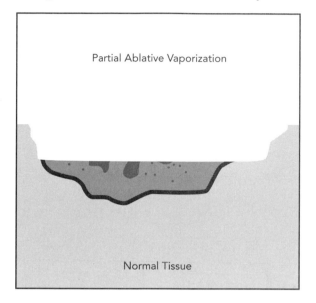

Figure 13. More Ablation of the Lesion by AV

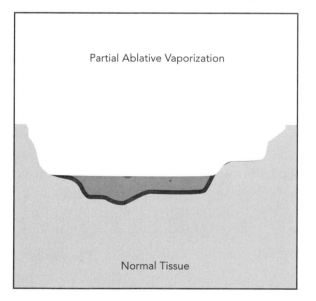

Figure 14. Normal Tissue Left After Complete AV

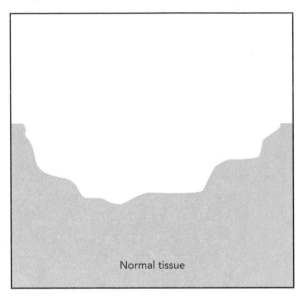

Normal tissue

The black line in Figure 10, which is the same as the white line in Figure 7, represents the last layer of cells vaporized with AV. This line of vaporized tissue is the same with either EV or AV. The only difference is that this line of cells is removed first with EV and, as I say, last with AV. The effect on the remaining adjacent layer of normal cells—the layer next to this line of vaporized tissue—is the same with each process. (Compare Figures 9 and 14.) The primary difference is that with AV, all the endometriosis and surrounding margin of tissue are vaporized, while with EV, a piece of tissue is physically removed.

You may hear people, even physicians, mistakenly say that the laser or Ablative (Area) Vaporization burns (coagulates) the tissue, and that Ablative Vaporization is not a good technique for removing endometriosis. The physics of heat and thermal energy tells us that those statements are incorrect. Vaporization hits a cell with energy that is so quick, intense, and precise, that the cell is eliminated, while the cell next to it is undamaged. There is virtually no conduction of heat, so the cells next to the last line of vaporized cells are not affected by the heat of vaporization.

Coagulation results from conduction of heat, which is when heat travels through the tissues, spreading from one cell to the next and melting the cellular proteins. Imagine putting your finger on a hot iron. The longer you leave it on the iron, the more severely you will be burned, because the heat is being conducted from the iron to your finger. In contrast, if you whip your finger through a candle flame quickly enough, you will not get burned, because the heat is not being conducted.

Coagulation (see Figure 15) burns just the top of the endometriosis and will usually result in incomplete removal, leaving the patient feeling the endometriosis has "grown back" in a short amount of time (months to a year or two).

Figure 15. Coagulation of Endometriosis

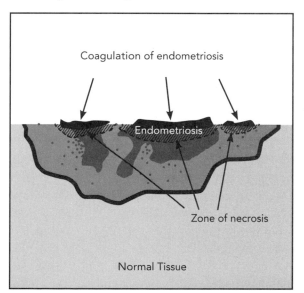

Instead of vaporization (EV or AV), many general OB/GYN surgeons try to remove endometriosis using coagulation. Cauterization, one of two types of coagulation, uses heat from an electrical current to cause coagulation; the other type, fulguration, uses high-frequency electrical current to burn and dry the surface of the tissue. Think of burnt toast or bacon. This is what the char of coagulation looks like. This zone of char is a problem for two reasons. First, the surgeon cannot tell if all the endometriosis has been burned, since it is just black char. Second, the char can prevent the coagulation from going deep enough to burn all the tissue. Additionally, some of the heat is conducted beyond the coagulation, spreading under the char, and it damages the surrounding tissue. This is called the zone of necrosis: the zone of death. Initially, the tissue looks fine, so, even if you could see it, you couldn't tell if there is a problem. But it is actually dead, and over the next couple of days, the tissue will turn black and die. This can be serious if part of a vital structure, such as the bowel, is destroyed. It could cause a massive infection that's deadly or requires a colostomy bag. For removal of endometriosis, coagulation simultaneously lacks the precision to remove all the endometriosis and spreads damaging levels of heat, causing unforeseen and unwanted damage to normal surrounding tissue.

Table 1 below lists surgical terms and their definitions to help you better understand the techniques by seeing them listed altogether.

Table 1. Surgical Terms

Ablative Vaporization	Vaporizing an area of cells, completely removing all the cells in that area (AV).
AV	Ablative Vaporization, also known as Area Vaporization
cauterization	Passing electrical current through tissue to cause coagulation. This is a type of electrical burn. It is derived from the Greek word kauterion, meaning "branding iron."
coagulation	Disruption of tissue by heat, causing denaturation and clumping of protein. This occurs at temperatures between 65 degrees centigrade and less than 100 degrees centigrade.
EV	Excisional Vaporization. The primary technique used in surgery to cut and excise tissue. EV is also the simpler and abbreviated form for TEL-V.
excision	Surgical removal or resection
fulguration	Drying tissue by high-frequency electrical current. The word is derived from the Latin meaning "sheet lightning."
Linear Vaporization	Vaporizing cells in a line, cutting the tissue. This results in Excisional Vaporization, or EV.
mechanical energy	Energy derived from physical force, such as muscles
ME	Mechanical Excision
TEL-V	Thermal Excision by Linear Vaporization, also known as EV or Excisional Vaporization.
thermal energy	Energy derived from a heat source
vaporization	The action or process of turning liquid or solid into vapor. This occurs at temperatures greater than 100 degrees centigrade.

Surgical Techniques: Wide Excision and Wide Ablative Vaporization

In the majority of endometriosis surgeries, excision (EV) is the only technique required. With our current technology, in certain limited cases, Ablative Vaporization can be used as a secondary tool. Wide excision (both mechanical and thermal) and wide Ablative Vaporization remove endometriosis from the body most effectively. Coagulation, including cauterization and fulguration, burns the endometriosis and leaves it in the body; this technique is ineffective. Table 2 shows the relationships between energy and technique.

Table 2. Energy and Surgical Techniques

Type of Energy	Effect of Energy	Surgical Technique
Mechanical	Cutting	Excision (removal)—good
Thermal	Cutting—Vaporization—Linear	Excision (removal)—good
Thermal	Vaporization—Ablative	Ablation (removal)—good
Thermal	Coagulation	Denature protein (burns tissue)—bad
Thermal	Cauterization	Denature protein (burns tissue)—bad
Thermal	Fulguration	Denature protein (burns tissue)—bad

Now that you understand the details of excision by EV and AV, let's talk a little about how a surgeon decides which of these surgical techniques is best for removing endometriosis.

Excision can be performed surgically in one of two ways: by mechanical excision (ME) or by Thermal Excision by Linear Vaporization (EV). Mechanical excision makes use of only the mechanical shearing force of scissors, without the aid of electrosurgery. It is rarely used in surgery today. EV uses electrosurgery, laser, or the harmonic scalpel to create the intense heat that results in vaporization. Almost all endometriosis surgeons use some variation of EV.

Both methods of excision (ME and EV) can quickly remove large amounts of tissue and provide tissue for a pathologist to examine under a microscope—two important positives. Neither method damages or alters the appearance of the underlying tissue. This is important, because whenever tissue is removed, the remaining underlying tissue must be assessed to determine if deeper disease is still present.

With our current technology, Ablative Vaporization should not be used as the primary or only means of removing endometriosis; it is acceptable in limited situations by surgeons who have the necessary surgical skills. One problem with our current surgical technology (including the CO_2 laser, electrosurgery, and other sources of thermal energy) is the small-spot size or area that is ablated (vaporized). This is great for cutting with EV, since it is very small and precise. But with AV, it is difficult to ablate large amounts of tissue. Think of it as trying to paint a room with a tiny brush. It could be done, but the reality is that it would be difficult to get a nice even coat.

In the future, if we have a technology that provides a larger-diameter laser beam, AV could be used by most surgeons to completely remove endometriosis. One laser company is currently developing a scanning laser laparoscope that could solve this problem, making Ablative Vaporization an option as a primary tool for treating Stage I and Stage II endometriosis. The scanning laser has a computer that controls the movement of the laser beam, moving it in a predetermined pattern to completely ablate a given area of tissue. It has the effect of providing a much larger spot, similar to having a larger brush with which to paint.

Ablative Vaporization can be performed with the carbon-13 CO_2 laser or through electrosurgery. The laser is the most precise surgical tool available for removing endometriosis. Because the packet of light energy is so intense and focused, there is very little conduction of heat and no coagulation, so there's virtually no thermal damage to the tissue left behind. (It does not burn tissue!) This allows the surgeon to remove the endometriosis layer by layer, and thus to be more precise than he or she could be using excision by EV. This is especially useful when working on vital structures, such as blood vessels, the bowel, or the ureter.

An example of an appropriate use of Ablative Vaporization is with endometriosis involving the small bowel, because this is like trying to remove chunks of dried glue from tissue paper with a pair of scissors, without damaging the tissue paper. A surgeon who uses only EV or ME excision may have to leave some endometriosis on the bowel or perform a segmental small bowel resection, because "the endometriosis was so extensive."

Ablative Vaporization is also the preferred technique when there is small, superficial endometriosis on the ovary or the fallopian tubes. In these cases, Ablative Vaporization does the job: the bowel, ovary, or fallopian tube is left in place, undamaged, and the endometriosis is completely removed.

The Five Rules for Correct Surgical Treatment of Endometriosis

1. Burning the endometriosis with coagulation or cauterization is bad. In all likelihood, some endometriosis will remain, and the patient's pain will persist or return rather quickly.

2. Excision is the preferred method of removing endometriosis. There is growing consensus among advanced laparoscopic surgeons and en-dometriosis experts that endometriosis should be removed by excision.

3. EV is the preferred method of excision. In performing excision, the vast majority of endometriosis experts are linear vaporizers. They use thermal energy to excise the endometriosis, through a technique known as thermal excision by linear vaporization (TEL-V or EV).

4. Ablative Vaporization is an acceptable secondary technique for removing small areas of endometriosis. While theoretically AV can produce the exact same results as EV, the laser beam produces such a small dot, it's hard to vaporize large amounts of tissue without missing some cells. When precise removal of a small area of endometriosis is required, wide Ablative Vaporization by a qualified surgeon can provide more precise removal of tissue and is an acceptable alternative to excision.

5. Use wide excision and wide Ablative Vaporization. It is important to remove a rim of normal tissue around the endometriosis to get rid of all the endometriosis, including microscopic disease.

EVE Procedure™

This is a term I coined to describe the correct surgical removal of endometriosis. EVE stands for **E**xcision and **V**aporization of **E**ndometriosis (also **E**xcisional **V**aporization of **E**ndometriosis). Most of the top endometriosis surgeons use the EVE Procedure™ to remove endometriosis. Even the advocates of excision only who use thermal energy are performing EV and thus using the EVE Procedure™. If EVE were used in all operating rooms during endometriosis surgery, there would be a lot less pain and suffering!

Robotic Surgery

Robotic surgery is really just a type of modified laparoscopic surgery. Many hospitals and some surgeons are marketing the da Vinci Robot (the only robot currently available) as providing more advanced surgery with better outcomes and a quicker return to work. Unfortunately, these claims do not specify what type of surgery they are comparing it to.

When comparing robotic surgery to the old type of surgery (laparotomy), which requires large incisions, the more advanced robotic surgery looks like an improvement. But, if they compared robotic surgery to traditional laparoscopic surgery, they couldn't make the same claims.

Robotic surgery is not less invasive than traditional laparoscopic surgery; it is actually more invasive resulting in a bigger cut, requiring more incisions in more visible areas on the body. Proponents of robotic surgery state it may offer an improved ability to dissect areas of endometriosis, but those proponents also admit a lack of evidence. As of 2012 no scientific studies show better outcomes for endometriosis patients treated with robotic surgery than with traditional laparoscopy.

The robot is just a different way of getting to the tissue. All the principles discussed previously regarding energy, excision, vaporization, and coagulation apply. Coagulating endometriosis with a robot is no better than coagulating endometriosis with the traditional laparoscopic approach. Wide excision of endometriosis is a very specific skill that surgeons must learn over time with practice and guidance from an experienced surgeon. While the robot can provide a different way of getting to the tissue, it cannot, in itself, provide a new surgical skill (performing wide excision) to the surgeon.

In my opinion, the biggest drawback to the da Vinci robot is the issue of cosmesis. Cosmesis in this situation refers to the ability to perform surgery without leaving visible scars, which is usually possible with traditional laparoscopy. With traditional laparoscopy, cosmesis is very possible since the location of the incisions—and thus scars—can be placed in an area that is well hidden (even by a small bikini) and not visible. In contrast, the da Vinci robot leaves quite a few clearly visible scars on the abdomen. The robot requires larger-sized incisions and at least one, and usually two, additional incisions, all located in the middle of the abdomen, leaving three or four clearly visible and relatively large scars. It is not the end of the world to have scars all over your abdomen, but why do it if you have another option?

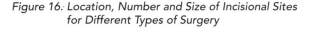

Figure 16. Location, Number and Size of Incisional Sites for Different Types of Surgery

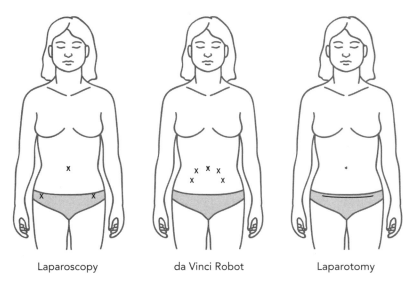

| Laparoscopy | da Vinci Robot | Laparotomy |

Without a clear advantage, one wonders both why so many hospitals and gynecologists are converting to the robot and how the use of robotic surgery may affect the quality of surgery provided to endometriosis patients. At this point, we do not have the information necessary to answer these questions. But we do have some information regarding hysterectomies and the robot. While hysterectomies are easier surgeries to perform than endometriosis surgery, we can use the hysterectomy information to help provide insight into how this might affect surgical treatment of endometriosis.

Basically there are three types of hysterectomy: abdominal, vaginal, and laparoscopic. Abdominal hysterectomy uses a big incision similar to a C-section, either low above the pubic bone or up and down between the pubic bone and the belly button. Vaginal hysterectomy is surgery done through the vagina, including removal of the uterus. Laparoscopic hysterectomy is performed with a laparoscopy through three small incisions.

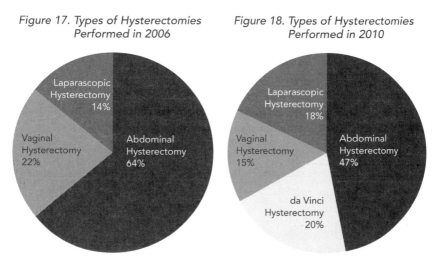

Figure 17. Types of Hysterectomies Performed in 2006

Laparascopic Hysterectomy 14%
Vaginal Hysterectomy 22%
Abdominal Hysterectomy 64%

Figure 18. Types of Hysterectomies Performed in 2010

Laparascopic Hysterectomy 18%
Vaginal Hysterectomy 15%
Abdominal Hysterectomy 47%
da Vinci Hysterectomy 20%

Recent data (private data, not from a peer-reviewed journal) confirms a shift in the types of hysterectomies performed in the United States.[57] The data in Figures 17 and 18 suggest that laparoscopic surgeons are continuing to perform non-robotic laparoscopic hysterectomies, while surgeons previously performing abdominal and vaginal hysterectomies are switching to robotic hysterectomies.

For 20 years following the first laparoscopic hysterectomy, only a small percentage of gynecologists (14 to 18 percent) were able to

---

57   Estimate based on 2008 Solucient data and ISI data on da Vinci hysterectomy procedures.

successfully perform this type of surgery. Yet in the five years since robotically assisted laparoscopic surgery was introduced, there has been a fairly rapid conversion from abdominal surgery to the robotic approach. It seems robotic surgery fills a gap in between laparoscopic surgery and the older laparotomy type of surgery. One has to ask what it is about laparoscopic surgery that seems to be so difficult for most surgeons, and what is the robot doing to help overcome this difficulty. The answer is spatial disorientation and reverse (or mirrored) movement.

One unspoken issue most gynecologists have with traditional laparoscopic surgery is what is known as spatial disorientation. When operating through a large incision during laparotomy, the surgeon looks directly through the opening in the body and performs the surgery with their hands. With laparoscopy, surgeons view their surgical movements on a monitor, which is in a completely different location and orientation from the tissue being operated on. The orientation (above/below, horizontal/vertical, left/right) of the actual surgery occurring in the patient from the surgeon's point of view varies throughout the procedure as well. To help visualize what this is like in surgery, think of a large salad bowl in a big box, and rather than looking at the bowl and inside of the box directly, it was displayed on a TV sitting on a table a few feet away. If you were standing next to it and had to clean every surface inside the bowl and box with a scrub brush and without moving either the bowl or the box, you would have to work on surfaces across from you, facing away from you, as well as up and down—only by watching what you are doing on the TV.

The second issue encountered in laparoscopic surgery is reverse (or mirrored) movement. Laparoscopic instruments are like sticks with scissor-like handles on one end that control differing shapes (for example graspers and scissors) that open and close on the other end. Because the instrument pivots around the abdominal wall, to move the instrument to the left while inside the body, the surgeon must move the outside end of the instrument to the right and vice versa. To move up inside the body requires outside movement down in the opposite direction. To continue the example above, rather than using the scrub brush directly to clean the bowl and inside of the box, attach the scrub brush to a stick going through the top of the box and move the stick on the outside of the box to clean the inside while watching the TV. Every movement you make with the stick is opposite and backward from the movement of the brush.

The robot does solve both the spatial disorientation and reverse movement problem. The surgeon sits at a console away from the patient looking through a viewfinder type of device at a virtual world in front of the surgeon just as if they were looking into the body through a big incision, with movements in the correct relative direction. This is the reason surgeons can now switch from an abdominal to a robotic approach, even if they are not comfortable with traditional laparoscopy.

I don't want to sound anti-robot because I am not. I have and do use the robot in select appropriate cases. Quite frankly, it is fun to use and it is much more comfortable sitting at a console working in the 3D virtual world of robotic surgery than the standing, bending, and twisting required when doing traditional laparoscopy. Like many things in life, robotic surgery has its advantages: 3D view, increased magnification, "wristed" instrument movement—and its disadvantages: delayed and restricted range of movement, inability to directly interact with the patient during surgery (important for adjusting the position of the uterus and bowel), lack of haptics (ability to feel touch including pressure or resistance), limitations in surgical tools and types of surgical energy, and more scars (lack of cosmesis). The robot is evolving and getting better all of the time. The current limitations will eventually be resolved with this evolution. Some type of computer and technologically assisted surgery will certainly become the standard type of surgery in the future. At this point in time, if a surgeon does not need the advantages of the robot, including help with spatial orientation, then the current disadvantages including cosmesis seem to preclude its adoption by the vast majority of endometriosis specialists. Perhaps I am an idealist, but I am compelled to do what I think is in my patients' best interest and treat them as I would want to be treated.

In my opinion as an advanced endometriosis surgeon, there is nothing I can do with the robot that I cannot do with traditional laparoscopy, and there are still a couple of significant disadvantages with the robot including limited types of surgical energy sources and inability of the surgeon to control the position of the uterus. It does seem the robot may allow a surgeon to use their laparotomy skills with the robot, even if they cannot perform them laparoscopically. Clearly, doctors who are going to provide surgical treatment of endometriosis, no matter what type of surgical approach they use, must be well trained to safely perform dissection and wide excision of endometriosis

After Surgery

When my team and I perform surgery, we make sure the patient is administered adequate pain medication, so that when she wakes up, she will feel the least amount of discomfort. Unlike many surgeons, I prefer to keep my patients in the hospital overnight after surgery. This enables them to use a pain-medication pump, which they can control for the most effective pain relief. Additionally, if needed, anti-nausea medication can be administered intravenously.

The next morning, we make sure the pain pills we've prescribed for post-operative pain management are working for the patient. We make sure her bladder is working properly, that she doesn't have nausea, that she has adequate pain relief. Then we send her home.

The first week, she probably isn't going to have to look at the clock to know when it's time for more pain meds. Some of my patients, however, have had such bad pain with endo, they wake up from surgery already feeling better. I find this amazing. How many people can understand that some women with endo are enduring pain every month that's worse than the pain after surgery?

Slowly she starts to recover. I don't want her to make any jerky moves that could tear muscle fibers when they're sore and bruised. I tell her to do any activities slowly and gently, easing back into her normal routine. During weeks two and three, she needs to take fewer pain meds and typically can go to work for a few hours or work from home. She's easily wiped out, though, sleeping a lot. Surgery takes a lot out of you.

By four to six weeks after surgery, she should be well recovered—and feeling better than she has in years. Recovery is a bit slower with wide excision than with surgery that coagulates a few lesions. Wide excision is a more involved surgery, though well worth the results.

We continue to see patients even after they recover, to make sure they get the comprehensive care they need: any supplements, medications, physical therapy, or other treatments dictated by their situation. While surgery can provide complete relief for some patients, many need to spend the next couple of months rebuilding their health. If the new, healthier habits and approach to living they've learned become a way of life, the future is bright.

The Well-informed Patient

I hope this chapter has helped you gain a better understanding of what to expect during surgical treatment of endometriosis. To summarize, I believe that good surgical techniques include the use of instruments that excise and vaporize, while using instruments that coagulate or cauterize the endo are bad surgical techniques. Cautery is required to seal any bleeders in all surgeries and is an appropriate use of this technique, even when vaporizing. Wide excision is the primary surgical technique in removing endometriosis laparoscopically; in many cases, it is the only method needed to remove all the endo safely. With more difficult or microscopic endo, wide Ablative Vaporization is an adjunct treatment that provides the precision necessary to remove it completely while leaving the normal tissue and vital structures intact. I call this the EVE (Excision and Vaporization of Endometriosis) Procedure™. The vast majority of endometriosis specialists use some variation of the EVE Procedure,™ even if they do not use this name.

I've gone into all this detail on surgical techniques because I believe you should be as informed as possible before you go into the operating room. As a group, women suffering from endometriosis can make a big difference in the care provided by the medical community, by demanding a level of expertise and excellence that will result in more effective treatment of their condition.

If all patients required their physicians to videotape their surgery, for instance, I believe the level of care would rise no matter what surgical technique is used. Video documentation of the surgery provides accountability and the facts. If a surgeon tells you that he or she does not have the equipment to videotape the procedure, you may want to think twice about proceeding. Good surgeons should be proud of their work and are glad for any and all to see the "masterpiece" they have created.

✿ ✿ ✿

"After years of being misdiagnosed, I was in so much pain I don't know how I held on. But the day came for the surgery that would improve my life. The surgery took two and a half hours. Barely awake afterwards, I slurred, "Was it endo?" My doctor verified that it was. As I was wheeled out, I said, "Twenty-one years. ..." My left ovary had been covered in endometriosis and stuck to my front abdominal wall, as well as to my bowels. It was a mess. No wonder the pain. Within one month, I felt completely better. No more pain! I joined the gym and started boxing boot camp. Heck, I even boxed during my period! It felt so good to be healed." —Lillyth

"My doctor estimated that the surgery would last three to four hours. It lasted over seven hours and was one of the worst cases he had ever seen. The endometriosis was adhered to the vaginal wall. It affected my appendix. My left ovary was gigantic, even bigger than my uterus. As I awoke, the surgical team put me at ease. They told me I was going to be okay. They told me that during the surgery, they had played the CD I'd recorded , which made me smile. Afterwards, I didn't need the prescription for Vicodin they gave me; the post-op pain was not that bad. I was home the next day. By the second week, the pain was COMPLETELY GONE. My period in April, before the surgery, was so painful. My period in May gave me NO CRAMPS. I have never had pain since. I smiled. I laughed. After a very long time, my life was back." (Note: the patient had a relaxation/positive affirmation CD she wanted us to play through her earphones during her surgery while she was asleep.)—I-Li

"My first surgery was at age 27, 14 years after my first episode of pain. The doctor found endometriosis everywhere and took out as much as she could. She told me there were only negligible amounts left, due to endometrial implants growing in very difficult areas that she didn't have the expertise to remove, and that I should have no residual pain from what was left in.

"Two years after my first surgery, I had surgery with a different doctor. Now I had two experiences to learn from. After the first surgery, the effects of the anesthesia were horrible; I was nauseated, and there were 10 young researchers standing around my bed. They sent me home the first day. With the second, I had a better experience with the anesthesia, was given anti-nausea medication, and my doctor took his time. He found that I had interstitial cystitis. The endometriosis was slowly inducing appendicitis. There was scar tissue around my gallbladder, but he saved my gallbladder. He found endometriosis around my ribs, ovaries, uterus, and colon, and he got it all, even the difficult areas of growth around my uterus that the first surgeon could not address. This time, I was not nauseated, and I stayed in the hospital overnight. My recovery took about six weeks. I had a little bit of post-op pain, but my underlying, constant pain was gone. But I was afraid of my period. To my amazement, it showed up with no warning and NO CRAMPING at all. I cried tears of joy." —Gabrielle

CHAPTER SEVEN

Pain and Pain Management

Dealing with the Pain of Endometriosis

Few medical conditions are as painful as endometriosis. What starts as painful periods usually becomes more intense and prolonged over time. Patients describe the pain as knifelike, burning, tearing, hot, sharp, and even worse than childbirth. What originates as cyclic pain becomes chronic pain. Women with endometriosis can experience dizziness, nausea, headaches, diarrhea, constipation, gastrointestinal distress, fatigue, and a general achy feeling—a sense of being completely depleted and out of sorts.

For some women with endo, the pain becomes severe and chronic enough that they can't make plans, because they don't know whether they will be curled up in a ball on the bed that day, trying to breathe through stabbing pain. The ongoing pain and disruption to everyday life can lead to despair and hopelessness, and the fear that you will never feel like yourself again. You start feeling isolated and alone, with nothing but pain for a (sometimes constant) companion.

And yet, we live in a culture in which "female pain" has been expected and seen as something women need to suffer through, because … they're women. People—including some doctors—are reluctant to talk about "female pain." It's only relatively recently that we've felt comfortable acknowledging menstrual pain, by, for instance, advertising over-the-counter drugs like Midol on TV.

Women who try to express what they're going through are too often accused of being complainers, hypochondriacs, or drug seekers. Sometimes there's even a whiff of blame: if the woman had just had children early enough, hadn't been so sexually active, had somehow taken better care of herself, or were a little tougher, she wouldn't be feeling such pain. Though none of those issues has any bearing on endo, the outrageous notion that somehow the woman brought it on herself still exists. On top of everything else, it is not uncommon for a woman to feel ashamed of her pain.

The frustration of not being heard or believed can be almost as excruciating as the pain itself. As one of my patients put it, "I sometimes wish my pelvis were a TV screen, so people could see what's going on inside." A woman with endo is often in a double bind: if she tries to describe or discuss her pain, she can be labeled as a chronic complainer; if she doesn't discuss it, people don't have a clue what she is going through. Either way, she is discouraged from seeking medical help.

Women with endometriosis often have to fight the medical system. They may have to fight to get their doctors to believe them and then treat them effectively. All too often they have to overcome the notion that their pain is more psychologically based than physical. They have to argue for coverage from insurance companies whose systems don't fit the complexity of their disease, which means it's often difficult for them to receive adequate coverage for the multiple medical treatments they need. After seeing thousands of women in debilitating pain, I want to tell you that if you have endometriosis, *your pain is real*, and it takes real courage for you to deal with it every day.

Stand Up for Your Pain

We've finally come to accept that stomach ulcers, another unseen illness, are real. It used to be thought that stomach ulcers were just a result of stress. We now know that a particular type of bacterial infection in the stomach causes the ulcers. We can create the same sort of awareness and understanding about endometriosis. If women with chronic pelvic pain and endo start challenging the myths and archaic attitudes, they will eventually teach people, including healthcare specialists, about the realities of this disease. Here are a few ways to do that:

- Don't blame yourself for your pain. Don't let yourself say or think, "If only I hadn't ..." or "If I were stronger. ..." You are not the cause of your pain.

- Educate the people in your life who need to understand what you're living with. Do it at a time when you can be unemotional, so that you can speak clearly and they can hear what you're saying. Communicate honestly and directly about your pain, but don't go on and on about it. Venting your frustration is usually counterproductive. People will tend to tune you out and think you are over-reacting.

- Find a support group for people in chronic pain, which can validate your experience, help you with coping strategies, and aid you in explaining your disease to others (see page 189 for a list of support groups). Chronic pain can rob you of your friends and support network. It helps to talk and even vent with people who really understand.

- Find the best treatment possible. If your doctor doesn't believe what you say about your pain, find another doctor. If your doctor will not provide you with adequate pain relief or refer you to a pain-management specialist, find another doctor. (A list of pain-management resources can be found in the Resources section on page 187.)

- Don't let anyone make you ashamed of taking the medication your doctor prescribes. Taking painkillers does not mean you are a drug addict. It means you need pain relief.

- Stand up for yourself with insurance companies and employers. Insist they acknowledge that your pain is real and that you need adequate treatment and support.

"I was in pain for 10 years. In a good month, I had a full week when I did not have pain. The majority of the time, I was in pain, and it was escalating. It was always around 5 out of 10. When my cycle came, it would hit 15 out of 10. Many doctors told me there was nothing wrong with me, but you can either be angry at the medical profession or you can decide, 'I'm tired of feeling like this, and I'm going to find somebody who understands.' One doctor told me, 'I've offered you hormones, and we're done here.' I said he should take a look inside; it didn't make sense. He said, 'Of course it doesn't make sense to you. How many years of medical school have you had?' I said, 'How many years have you been a woman?'" —Kelli

Why Does Endometriosis Hurt So Much?

Endometriosis acts like menstrual tissue in that it builds up through-out the month and then sheds. The problem is, unlike menstrual tis-sue, the endometriosis has nowhere to go. It stays in the body and causes inflammation throughout the pelvic region. The endometrial cells themselves release inflammatory chemicals (prostaglandins and histamines). All that inflammation irritates the pain receptors.

Organs stuck to one another with scar tissue may tug every time you move. When endometriosis starts eating into tissues or organs, the pain receptors in those areas will react. The pelvic region is full of inflamed blisters that hurt every time they rub against other tissue; when, like blisters popping, the endo ruptures, that sends out even more inflammatory chemicals, which further irritates the pain recep-tors. Repeated inflammation may make the pain receptors even more sensitive. It's a vicious cycle that gets ever more painful with time. The pain is often worst during menstruation, when hormone levels are changing, the endometriosis can be bleeding, and the tissues in the pelvis expand, which stretches and strains those pain receptors.

Endometriosis is a complicated disease, and there's a lot we don't know about why the pain is so deep and diffuse. Several studies have shown that the deeper the lesions, the more pain they cause, probably because they directly irritate the pelvic nerves.[58] There's also speculation that scar tissue can increase the level of pain by limiting the blood supply to the nerves.

Recent studies have shown that endometriosis creates new nerve fibers. Researchers at Florida State University, for instance, found that rats with endometriosis grow nerve supplies that communicate with the brain. These nerves probably grow along with the blood vessels that nourish the endometriosis. The researchers, who reproduced these findings in human tissue, speculate that the new nerve cells may be a reason endometriosis often shows up with other, seemingly unrelated conditions, such as irritable bowel syndrome and interstitial cystitis. When the new nerve supply sends signals to the central nervous system, the signals interact with messages from the other organs in the region that the brain interprets as pain. The wide variety in the nerve supply to endometriosis may explain why the severity of pain varies from one patient to another.[59]

Endometriosis Classification and Pain

It's important to point out that the pain doesn't correlate with how "serious" the disease is, based on how we chart the levels, or stages, of endometriosis. These stages were developed by the American Society for Reproductive Medicine, mostly to predict infertility. The stages indicate the size, depth, and extent of endometriosis, as well as how much scar tissue is involved. Stage I (minimal) is described as mostly showing superficial lesions. Stage II (mild) also shows some deeper lesions in the pelvis. Stage III (moderate) has all of the above plus either deep endometriosis in the ovary or ovaries (endometrioma cysts, or chocolate cysts) or scar tissue of the ovaries and/or fallopian tubes. Stage IV (severe) usually has all of the problems of Stage III endo plus obliteration of the posterior cul-de-sac, which is the space normally

---

58   Koninckz PR, Meuleman C, Demeyere S, Lesaffre E, Cornellie FJ. Suggestive evidence that pelvic endometriosis is a progressive disease, whereas deeply infiltrating endometriosis is associated with pelvic pain. *Fertility and Sterility*. 1991;(4)55:759-765.

59   Berkley KJ, Rapkin AJ, Papka RE. The pains of endometriosis. *Science*. 2005;308(5728):1587-1589.

present behind the uterus containing the bowel, ovaries, and fallopian tubes. With Stage IV endo, it is filled up with endometriosis and scar tissue gluing all of the above structures together.

I have seen many patients with Stage IV endometriosis who are in less pain than patients with Stage I or Stage II. It's a well-known fact that the stages indicate nothing about the level of pain a woman is experiencing. (They don't predict her level of fertility, either.) Clearly, there is need for a classification system that correlates with the severity of pain and level of fertility associated with endometriosis.

Pelvic pain is a complex condition that can be the result of any of numerous underlying problems. Often, the intensity of the pain is the culmination of several of these conditions existing at the same time. Endometriosis is one of the leading causes of pelvic pain. If endo was the main cause of your pain and you've had good surgery, it's possible that much or all of your pain was alleviated. But because of the nature of endometriosis and the co-conditions, some pain may persist. It's important to understand different kinds of pain, and what to do to be as comfortable as possible. Even after surgery for endometriosis and adhesions, you may need ongoing pain management to treat your other conditions.

Types of Pain

There are three basic types of pain. Nociceptive pain is associated with a healthy, normally functioning nervous system. Neuropathic pain and centralized pain are the results of an abnormally functioning nervous system.

Nociceptive pain Nociceptors are the nerve endings that sense irritation or injury; when they're activated, they transmit pain signals to the brain. It's often a cause-and-effect kind of response: you put your hand on a hot stove, and your pain receptors shriek, "Take that hand away!" This is considered healthy pain, because it alerts you that something is wrong. Usually the pain is limited to one place and doesn't have an all-over achy, throbbing quality. You feel nociceptive pain when you have such injuries as a bump, bruise, burn, bite, or broken bone. Visceral pain is nociceptive pain that involves the internal organs. That kind of pain tends to radiate.

But normally any kind of nociceptive pain is of fairly short duration. It usually responds well to painkillers, and when the damaged tissue heals, the pain goes away. This is the simple kind of pain we're all familiar with. Unfortunately, as with everything else about endometriosis, the pain involved with this disease can be complicated.

Neuropathic pain Pain is much more difficult to treat when it becomes neuropathic, meaning that it affects the peripheral nerves and central nervous system. When that happens, these nerves send out pain signals even when the pain stimulus is not present. This occurs when the pain has been chronic. For instance, if you put vice grips, or locking pliers, on your finger, you will feel nociceptive pain: ouch, that hurts. When the vice grip is removed, the pain will go away fairly quickly. If you leave the vice grips on for a year, however, your finger will never be the same; it will always be tender. Even though you've finally removed the pliers, and the initial, nociceptive cause of the pain is gone, the pain will remain. The pain is now neuropathic.

The same thing can happen with endometriosis. The constant alarm from pain signals starts to damage the alarm system itself. Problems with the immune system—and the inflammatory chemicals released—can make the pain receptors even more sensitive. In endometriosis with neuropathic pain, the entire pelvic region starts to hurt. Some studies have shown that if any part of the bowel, bladder, or reproductive organs has pain, it reduces the pain threshold for the others. Prolonged pain turns into something much less specific and, as I say, much more difficult to treat.

Remember, endometriosis is not the only cause of pelvic pain, so surgery does not always fix everything. (About one-third of my patients get complete relief from surgery, although some 90 percent find their pain lessened after surgery.) Women who have had long-term pelvic pain may continue to feel some soreness and tenderness because of neuropathic pain. This is another reason to get effective treatment as soon as possible. The longer you leave the pain untreated, the more likely it is that neuropathic pain will develop, and the more difficult it will be to treat it.

Centralized pain When the pain system is overloaded with constant pain signals, the system itself starts acting like a nerve ending, shooting pain throughout the body. It's like someone turned up the volume on the pain system. Women with this type of pain, such as those with fibromyalgia, are sensitive to the slightest stimuli; even a little touch can feel very painful to them. Since their whole body is oversensitized, women with centralized pain usually need ongoing medical treatment and pain management.

Pain with Sex

Pain with sex (the medical term is dyspareunia) is one of the most common symptoms of endometriosis, and one of the most frustrating. Most women are upset not only because they aren't able to feel sexually satisfied but because they are unable to give their partner the pleasure they'd like to provide. It can cause emotional distress for both parties and, needless to say, can be extremely stressful on a relationship. Men may become frustrated that a once-satisfying sex life has evolved into a situation that is uncomfortable or painful for their partner and unfulfilling for both of them.

That's one of the reasons I like to have the patient's spouse or partner in my office, too, so that he or she can better understand why the woman is reluctant to have sex.

As with pelvic pain in general, pain with sex is not always caused solely by endometriosis. There can be many other causes and, often, several different reasons. All the problems need to be identified, and a treatment plan put into place for each, to get the best results.

For example, the area around the opening of the vagina, the vestibule, can be so tender that a light touch with a Q-tip can feel like getting stabbed with a knife. This is usually a result of vestibulitis, a form of vulvodynia. (For more information on these conditions, you can visit the websites found in the Resources section.)

Another condition that can make sex unbearable is pelvic-floor muscle spasm. Just under the skin is a series of muscles that extend from the pubic bone to the tailbone; when these muscles go into severe spasm, it can cause some of the worst pain imaginable. Often, the muscular contractions of orgasm make the pain worse.

Pelvic-floor spasm is common in women who have had pain in the pelvic area for a long time. We all naturally tense up against pain. Without realizing it, most women with pelvic pain are clenching their pelvic muscles, and this can go on for months and years. This condition will typically not resolve until the source of the pain is removed and then will usually require treatment from a highly specialized pelvic-floor physical therapist. (Your average physical therapist has no idea how to treat this condition.) Usually women, these therapists have devoted their practice to helping patients with pelvic pain, working internally through the vagina to strengthen and relax the muscles causing the pelvic spasms. Rarely, the muscles are in too much spasm for physical therapy to work. In such cases, we can use Botox to relax the muscles, and then follow up with physical therapy.

The pudendal nerves, which are located about halfway up the vagina at the three o'clock and nine o'clock positions, can become very sore, and the pain can be felt anywhere from the clitoris past the vaginal area and into the rectum. Low hormone levels and infections can also cause vaginal pain.

The bladder lies along the front of the vagina. Painful bladder conditions such as interstitial cystitis can cause pain with sex, as can endometriosis, adhesions (scar tissue), adenomyosis, fibroids, and ovarian cysts. If the uterus is tipped back, it can be hit during intercourse and cause pain (the medical term for that is collisional dyspareunia). Varicose (swollen and twisted) veins in the pelvis, pelvic congestion, and ovarian vein varicosity can cause painful intercourse.

Women with dyspareunia describe sex as a deep stabbing or jabbing pain, typically saying it feels as if her partner is hitting something that really hurts. What's causing the pain is the stretching and pulling of endometrial implants that are located just behind the vagina and lower uterus, in the area known as the posterior cul-de-sac. Some women feel pain with deep penetration; for others, even touching the vagina or clitoris can be painful. Some women feel pain only while having intercourse; for some, the pain lingers afterward. Others feel okay during sex only to experience severe pain or burning for hours or days afterwards.

Even when the pain disappears once the endo is removed, it isn't easy to go right back to having sex as if it was never an excruciating experience. It usually takes time for a woman to adjust to the idea of having sex again, because it was so painful before. For both patient and partner, it takes patience and a willingness to go slowly to get back to a satisfying sex life. Some of my patients have benefitted a great deal from seeing a sex therapist.

I suggest to a patient that when she feels the time is right, it's best to be in a position of control. She should tell her partner to lie back and relax and let her take a position on top. That way she can control the depth of penetration and the degree of activity. If there is a tender area, she can move so that he is not pushing on that area. She can slow down or stop.

Apart from good surgery, two things can help couples who are dealing with painful intercourse. The first is communication. Let's face it; most of us are a little squeamish about discussing sex, even with our intimate partner. We'd rather just do it, not talk about it. We may get as far as "I like this" or "Please do that," but communicating honestly and directly about painful sex is beyond the comfort level for many of us.

You may need to start talking when you're not in the middle of making love, making each other understand the nature of the pain and how it affects you emotionally. So many issues can come up: fear of not feeling attractive or sexy anymore, guilt about not satisfying your partner, worry that the problems with sex will cause your partner to find someone else to have sex with or your relationship to fail, fear of rejection. In this scenario, both people in the couple need to be heard. Your spouse or partner may say he feels frustrated or resentful about not being able to have sex, that he's worried about hurting you, that *he* feels rejected.

I'm not saying this is going to be easy. You may need to seek the help of a counselor or sex therapist to deal with these complicated issues. (See chapter ten.) Once you've been able to talk about these things when you're not in the heat of the moment, then I hope you can start communicating more during sex, being clear about what is uncomfortable and what might be a nice alternative. So that you can feel good when having sex, it's important to speak up when something hurts and you do not just suffer through. You don't want to avoid sex because you find it's uncomfortable to say what's going on for you.

Don't forget that sexual intercourse is only one kind of sex. There's a lot more on the menu if you're willing to do a little exploration. If you're open to trying, explore other ways to give your partner pleasure: oral sex, different positions, touching him even when you don't want to be touched sexually, mutual masturbation. You may have to avoid certain days of the month. You may end up doing a lot more kissing and cuddling than you used to.

These emotional and sexual issues are difficult for both women with endo and their partners. But I want my patients to feel good in every aspect of their lives. I think it's as important to heal the emotional and sexual pain as any other type of pain, because they are all interconnected. If you feel positive and sexy, that will reverberate throughout your entire being, and you will feel healthier. For that reason, I often recommend that my patients seek support beyond the medical office. (See chapters eight, nine, and ten.)

> "I have a really great guy who understands me. He's wonderful and gentle; he crawled into my hospital bed and held my hand. He understands when sex is painful, or I'm tired and don't feel well, and I'm very grateful for that. I had a relationship that fell apart because sex was painful. He didn't bother going to my doctor's appointments with me, so he didn't understand the illness, and he just thought I was crazy. If you're married and you have endo, you need to bring your husband along to the meetings with the specialist, so that he understands you have to embrace a certain lifestyle and change things a bit." —Kathleen

Pain Management

As with every other facet of endometriosis treatment, pain must be approached from the perspective of the whole patient. My approach is to create individual programs to help alleviate each patient's pain. These programs might include surgery, treatment of bladder conditions, food elimination, physical therapy, nerve blocks, hormonal medications, supplements, non-narcotic pain medications, narcotic pain medications, and mind-body stress reduction. Some patients have good results with chiropractic treatment, craniosacral therapy, or acupuncture. A board-certified pain-management physician can help in certain cases, especially when interventional pain management (pain pumps and catheters) is needed.

Once we have a comprehensive treatment plan, we stay alert to what is working and what is not, so that we know what to continue and what to stop. The goal is to get rid of the pain completely. That's a realistic possibility in many cases, and it happens with a good portion of our patients. Not all patients become pain-free, and often a more realistic goal is to reduce the pain enough that a patient who hasn't been able to function normally can begin to do the things she wants and needs to do. The pain may still be a nuisance, but it will not control her life.

Many patients have pain so severe, they need narcotic pain relief. It may be for only a couple days each month; it may be for chronic severe pain with breakthrough acute pain—that is, when it hurts all the time but sometimes hurts even more. Not all doctors, however, believe in using narcotic painkillers to treat what is known medically as "chronic nonmalignant pain," or long-term, severe pain not caused by cancer. These doctors are afraid their patients may abuse the pain meds. Some argue that over time, narcotics can actually make the pain worse, and that these patients will need more and more pain meds to get the same results. While this is a real concern, in my experience such patients are very rare exceptions. The overwhelming majority of patients do not want pain meds; they want relief from intense pain.

California has a comprehensive pain-prescription monitoring program, whereby a doctor can check every prescription filled by his or her patients in the state to make sure the patient is not getting narcotic painkillers from other doctors, too—double-dipping, as it were. In our office, we're very conscientious. We have a pain-narcotic contract with each patient that specifies all the things she can and can't do if she's going to be taking prescription-narcotic pain medications. Our entire staff meets once a month to discuss our patients who are taking narcotic pain meds. Every once in a while, unannounced, we ask these patients to give us a urine sample for a drug screen. Patients who need long-term treatment have to see a board-certified pain-management physician once a year.

We help our patients get the pain relief they deserve, in a supportive environment. Physicians take an oath to do no harm. From my perspective, ignoring a patient's pain and not helping is doing harm.

Pain-management Treatments

Dealing with pain can involve taking prescription or nonprescription drugs, as well as other approaches.

- Acetaminophen or Tylenol can be used alone or in combination with other pain medications. The maximum daily dose of acetaminophen, from whatever source—and it is in a lot of over-the-counter medications—is 4,000 mg. Check all your over-the-counter and prescription drugs for acetaminophen, and make sure you are not taking more than that amount each day. If you're taking acetaminophen over a long period of time, 2,600 mg a day is a more reasonable dose. Taking too much acetaminophen can damage your liver and even result in death.

- Non-steroidal anti-inflammatory drugs (NSAIDS), such as ibuprofen (Advil, Motrin), naproxen sodium (Aleve), and prescription NSAIDS, are generally used to suppress inflammation and treat mild pain. They vary in their potency and in how long they act. NSAIDS work by blocking the enzymes that make prostaglandins, which are chemicals that can cause inflammation and pain. Since prostaglandins also protect the stomach and support blood clotting, long-term use of NSAIDS can cause ulcers in the stomach and promote bleeding. NSAIDS generally work best if they're started before the pain begins. One trick with bad menstrual cramps is to take Motrin around the clock, 600 mg every six hours, starting two days prior to the worst pain. This can reduce the amount of both pain and bleeding. With ibuprofen, the maximum dose is 2,400 mg per day.

- Narcotics include short-acting opiates—such as hydrocodone (Norco, Vicodin, and Lortab), oxycodone (Percocet, Endocet, OxyIR), hydromorphone (Dilaudid), demerol, and fentanyl (Actiq lollipops)—and long-acting opiates, such as long-acting morphine (MS Contin), long-acting oxycodone (Oxycontin), and long-acting fentanyl (Duragesic skin patch). These drugs work by slowing down or stopping signals from the nerves to the brain via the central nervous system. Short-acting opiates are given alone, for acute or short-term pain, or with long-acting narcotics, for breakthrough or more intense pain in patients who suffer from chronic pain. In those cases, the patient takes the long-acting narcotics two or three times a day for baseline pain relief, and the short-acting pain meds when needed, as determined by the pain level.

- Pain pumps: Patients requiring long-term treatment may use implantable pain-management devices, what we call intrathecal drug delivery. Here, a small pump surgically placed under the skin of the abdomen delivers medication through a catheter to the area around the spinal cord, like an epidural during childbirth. With this approach, the patient gets relief with a smaller dose than normally used with oral medication.

- Spinal cord stimulators (also know as dorsal column stimulators) have an effect similar to pain pumps. These are small catheters, usually implanted along the spinal cord, that send out a low electrical current that cancels out the pain signal. A little generator box goes under the skin, usually in the abdominal area.

- Trigger-point injections, or nerve blocks: Patients who have abdominal-wall or pudendal-nerve pain can benefit from injections of numbing medicine into painful areas or overly sensitive nerves. This should provide temporary relief; in some cases, it can result in prolonged relief. Pain-management physicians can perform blocks in other parts of the body, as medically indicated, as well.

- Radiofrequency Ablation (RFA): Patients who feel only temporary relief with nerve blocks can get prolonged relief (three to six months) with RFA. This procedure uses sound waves to "stun" the nerve. We don't understand exactly how it works, but it does work and it is safe.

Addiction Issues

There's a social stigma around taking narcotics. Many patients (or their loved ones) are worried they'll become addicted. But there's a difference between physical dependence and addiction.

If you take enough narcotics long enough, you will become physically dependent: quit taking them suddenly, and you'll experience physical withdrawal. This does not mean that patients taking narcotics have a craving to take the drug. Patients who are in pain do not get high from the narcotics; the narcotics help reduce the pain to tolerable levels. There is no craving for narcotic pain meds. However, if a patient who's been taking narcotics for a long time has surgery that eliminates her pain, she can't just shout, "Hallelujah" and throw the drugs down the toilet. If she does, she's going to have withdrawal symptoms. Since her body has adapted to the narcotics, she has to taper off slowly, taking an ever-decreasing dose until she is completely off the narcotics. This process can take weeks or months, but it's rarely difficult to get off them.

The National Institute on Drug Abuse, a division of the National Institutes of Health, defines addiction as a chronic relapsing brain disease that is characterized by compulsive drug seeking and use, despite harmful consequences. In the case of addicted individuals, they are taking narcotics for reasons other than relief of their physical pain. An example of an addicted individual using narcotics inappropriately would be someone who is having a bad day and takes a Vicodin to help relieve a high degree of anxiety and stress. The vast majority of my patients don't take narcotics for reasons other than relief of physical pain, and they do not exhibit addictive behavior. In fact, studies conducted in burn units have shown that if a patient does not have prior addiction issues, the likelihood of problems with addiction to the narcotics taken for pain from the burns is very, very low. If you're in severe pain, you need and deserve effective pain relief, and sometimes that means taking narcotics.

CHAPTER EIGHT

Treating the Whole Patient: A New Paradigm

Healing involves a lot more than getting rid of disease. We are coming to a point in medicine where we finally realize that becoming healthy means more than treating a particular symptom or disease. Treating illness doesn't mean fixing just one part of the machine; we are complex beings, not component parts. We can't really speak of all our organ systems separately, or even of our "mind" apart from our "body," because they are interconnected; they are one. So to effectively treat endometriosis, we have to understand the bigger picture of a patient's well-being, and support her in all the ways that affect her health: lifestyle, environmental factors, relationships, ways of thinking, spirit, and attitude. We want to optimize her overall health.

Traditional Western medicine, however, has evolved primarily into a disease-management system, treating one particular symptom, one specific disease. Modern medicine does provide an amazing range of prescription medications, as well as high-tech procedures and surgeries that, while very expensive, provide fairly effective management of disease symptoms. I am grateful we have all these treatments, but I believe that to truly heal a patient, we have to change the way we think. We need a paradigm shift in the culture of medicine, to a more comprehensive approach to health and disease. In short, we need to treat the whole person.

Jon Kabat-Zinn, PhD, professor of medicine emeritus at the University of Massachusetts Medical School, in Worcester, pioneered the field of mind-body practices in medicine. He is the founding executive director of the Center for Mindfulness in Medicine, Health Care, and Society and the founder and former director of its renowned Stress Reduction Clinic. I recommend his book, *Full Catastrophe Living: Using the Wisdom of Your Body and Mind to Face Stress, Pain, and Illness* to my patients. In this book, he explains the importance of thinking in terms of wholeness and interconnectedness—about paying attention to the interactions of mind, body, behavior, and circumstances in treating chronic disease. "Science will never be able fully to describe a complex dynamic process such as health, or even a relatively simple chronic disease," he writes, "without looking at the functioning of the whole organism and not restricting itself to an analysis of parts and components, no matter how important that may be as well."[60]

In Western medicine, we've been taught to think of diseases as individual, discrete problems, with a particular set of symptoms. But the longer I practice, the more I see that other systems are often involved. Endometriosis is too complicated a condition to fit into the simple one-disease management method of Western medicine.

As I've said so often in these pages, the only way to treat endometriosis successfully is to remove it surgically, with wide excision. If you start a patient on other treatments to improve her overall health, that's fine; but as long as the endo remains, it'll be like driving with the emergency brake on. You have to remove the endometrial implants before you can really get anywhere. That's just the first step, though. Lack of disease does not equal a healthy body.

Many of the patients I see come in with a number of symptoms that may or may not be classically related to endometriosis but surely affect their overall health. Often, endometriosis is clustered with problems such as interstitial cystitis, insulin resistance, hypothyroidism, allergies and autoimmune diseases, food and environmental sensitivities, fibro-

60   Kabat-Zinn J. *Full Catastrophe Living: Using the Wisdom of Your Body and Mind to Face Stress, Pain, and Illness.* 15th ed. New York, NY: Bantam Dell; 1990:151.

myalgia, chronic fatigue syndrome, eczema, vaginal yeast infections, and Lyme disease, to name a few.[61] A 1998 survey of 3,680 members of the Endometriosis Association found that women with endometriosis had higher rates of hypothyroidism, rheumatoid arthritis, allergies, and asthma, among other medical problems.[62]

Because these other conditions so often co-exist with endometriosis, in addition to whatever medical treatment or surgery I do, I make sure that the patient's underlying metabolic system is in balance; that her digestive, immune, and hormonal systems are functioning optimally; that she's exercising and eating well. The better the patient's overall health, the easier it is to address all the underlying issues.

Functional Medicine

Endometriosis is considered a chronic disease, meaning that it develops over years; cancer, diabetes, and heart disease are other chronic diseases. Unlike food poisoning, the flu, or a broken bone, chronic disease usually results from an imbalance in the underlying physical systems. This underlying dysfunction not only can increase the risk of developing endometriosis; it can also show up as one of the chronic diseases I mentioned above.

This is why, in addition to surgery and traditional medication, I often take an approach to treatment that is called functional medicine.[63] This is a philosophy of treatment that treats the whole patient. It acknowledges that every patient is different, and that one aspect of that individuality is biochemical (how people function metabolically). Functional medicine is personalized for the patient and deals with the underlying causes of serious chronic disease. It focuses on "patient health," not "disease management," which means that I am interested

---

61 Barrier BF. Immunology of Endometriosis, Clinical Obstetrics and Gynecology, 2010;53(2):397-402.

62 Sinaii N, Cleary SD, Ballweg ML, Nieman LK, Stratton P High rates of autoimmune and endocrine disorders, fibromyalgia, chronic fatigue syndrome and atopic diseases among women with endometriosis: a survey analysis. Human Reproduction. 2002;17(10):2715–2724.

63 For more information on functional medicine, visit http://www.functionalmedicine.org

not only in the absence of disease in my patient but also in optimizing how all the underlying systems function in the body.

The old view of disease is that of one symptom, one disease, and one pharmaceutical drug to treat the symptom. The new paradigm considers that the human body functions as a web, a variety of systems connected to one another rather than functioning autonomously, with no effect on the rest of the body. Instead of focusing on just one symptom (which may be 10 or 20 steps from the original problem), we look at the entire system for imbalances that underlie these disease conditions. These imbalances are affected by genetic and epigenetic or environmental factors:

- Diet and nutrition
- Exercise
- Trauma
- Environmental toxins
- Infectious agents
- Emotions, attitude, and spirit: the mind-body connection

How an individual responds to all these factors depends on her genetic predispositions, her attitude, as well as her unique physiological processes, such as how her cells communicate and transform food into energy. Imbalances in these systems can affect hormones, the immune system, inflammation, metabolism, and detoxification, as well as the digestive, absorptive, and microbiological systems. Functional medicine looks at treating chronic diseases by intervening at many levels to address these core imbalances.

When there is an underlying disorder in several systems, an initial trigger—something that chronically stresses the body, such as an inflammatory diet or environmental toxins—may start the decline in health. Then other symptoms follow in a kind of cascade. The decline in the functionality of multiple organ systems causes an overall decline in the person's health.

The different systems involved can include the gastrointestinal system and its effect on the immune system; the endocrine system (which includes the various hormones released by the body: estrogen, progesterone, androgens, thyroid, growth hormone, and the stress hormone, cortisol); the nervous system; many aspects of the immune system; and possibly even the coagulation system. In its worst form, the underlying, multisystem dysfunction causes such low body function that performing even routine tasks becomes nearly impossible. I've certainly seen many patients in that state.

Successful treatment of these multisystem problems requires a comprehensive, sustained approach: correcting one system, then another, then another, until the patient begins to regain her health. It is not an easy process, nor is it always successful. Hopefully, as we gain more understanding of multisystem diseases, along with better diagnostic tests and more effective treatment, patients will see improved prognoses. With better understanding will come more acceptance of multifunctional therapies.

Common Underlying Health Problems with Endo

Let's take a look at some of the underlying processes that can affect overall health and thus endometriosis.

Bowel Function

The bowel, or gastrointestinal, tract is an extremely complicated system, with many functions beyond simple digestion. A healthy GI tract is necessary for good immune function. It is a delicate ecosystem, easily put out of balance by environmental factors, including antibiotics and an unhealthy diet. Restoration of optimal function is a crucial building block in the foundation of health. Some patients benefit from the 4R program: **R**emove toxins, **R**eplace missing factors, **R**epair the lining of the bowel, and **R**einoculate with probiotics. Probiotics are the good healthy bacteria, medically known as commensal bacteria. These friendly bacteria aid in digestion and are necessary for healthy bowel function. I recommend that patients take a good-quality probiotic (I prefer to use refrigerated probiotics).

Immune Response

While we do not completely understand the cause of endometriosis, an immune dysfunction may be involved in both the cause and some symptoms of the disease. Immune dysfunction means that the immune system is underactive—not doing its job—on one hand and overactive, on the other hand. Most women have some retrograde menstruation, or a backward flow of menstrual tissue, up through the fallopian tubes, in the pelvic area. For most women, the immune system usually works properly; it goes in and destroys that stray tissue, and the woman doesn't develop endometriosis. Obviously, this is not the case for women with endo, who may also have overactive immune systems, with an increased incidence of sensitivities, allergies, and autoimmune disease, such as Hashimoto's thyroiditis, which can lead to hypothyroidism.

Inflammation

Inflammation is the process by which the body's white blood cells, immune cells, and antibodies protect us from infection and foreign substances, such as bacteria and viruses. But sometimes the immune system triggers an inflammatory response when there are no foreign substances to fight. Endometriosis is a disease involving an inflammatory response.

Three examples follow of what can happen in the immune system with an inflammatory response:

- *Prostaglandins* These are compounds found in tissues that stimulate nerve cells. They swell the blood at the injured site, producing swelling and tenderness—signaling a problem by causing pain. With inflammation, there is too much of the prostaglandin E2, which increases aromatase activity, creating too much estrogen.

- *Cytokines* Produced by cells throughout the body, these hormones also modulate the immune system. Studies have shown that women with endometriosis have dysregulated cytokine production, which means there's a problem with the substances produced by the cells of the immune system. A subclass called leukotrienes calls off the immune response before it destroys outlying healthy cells and tissue; if these hormones are overactive, they cause an inflammatory response to endometrial tissue.

- *Histamines* These are the chemicals responsible for the itchy nose, watery eyes, and rash that can indicate an allergic reaction.

Because it is affected by foods we eat, inflammation is one area in which we can keep endometriosis in check after surgery. Nutritionists agree that SAD—the Standard American Diet, full of saturated fats and processed sugars and low in fruits and vegetables—tends to increase inflammation. One of the reasons we so often see food allergies with endometriosis is that both are related to inflammation. (More on this in the nutrition section, below).

Estrogen Dominance

As we've seen, estrogen is the key hormone promoting the growth of endometriosis. Estrogen dominance refers to an imbalance of estrogen in the system, which can lead to many problems: premenstrual tension (PMS), excessive or painful periods, fibroid uterine tumors, cervical dysplasia, ovarian cysts, mid-life obesity, lupus, breast cancer—and endometriosis.

Xenoestrogens—chemicals that can provoke or mimic estrogen—can be found in pesticides, plastics, deodorants, toothpaste, sunscreen, even some food preservatives. The list of xenoestrogens in our environment is long. (As of 2011, more than 500 scientific papers have been written on xenoestrogens, 211 on environmental xenoestrogens alone.)

Another cause of estrogen dominance is the enzyme called aromatase, which I discussed in chapter six. This enzyme is found in endometriosis itself, causing the disease to produce more estrogen. Chronic inflammation can increase aromatase activity.

Estrogen dominance also occurs when the estrogen is metabolized unfavorably. We've already seen how estrogen, when detoxified, or eliminated from the body, gets broken down in the liver into "good" or "bad" estrogen. Estrogen metabolized into 2-OH Estradiol or 2-OH Estrone (good estrogen) seems to be safely eliminated from the body. It's the estrogen metabolized into 16a-OH Estrone that seems to be the problem: with endometriosis, as with cancer and other diseases related to estrogen, there is too much of this "bad" estrogen. A few studies have shown that toxins such as dioxin stimulate metabolism of the bad estrogen. Premarin, the commercial name for estrogen from horse urine, which is sometimes prescribed for symptoms of menopause, seems to be preferentially metabolized as bad estrogen. It has been found to increase the risk of breast cancer.

Some nutrients—one is diindolylmethane, or DIM; another is vitamin D—can help break down the estrogen into "good" estrogen. These can be found in cruciferous vegetables. So eat your broccoli! (See page 160 for the exception.)

Insulin Resistance

When you eat, the food is broken down into glucose, the simple sugar that is the body's main source of energy. As the food goes into the blood, it causes blood-glucose levels to rise. The pancreas releases the hormone insulin to help the cells take in and use the glucose, thus keeping the blood-sugar level from getting too high. For some people, the insulin system does not work well from the time of birth, predisposing them to insulin resistance and weight gain from an early age. Both insulin levels and blood-sugar levels are higher in people with insulin resistance.

Not surprisingly, a diet high in refined carbohydrates and sugar will cause the pancreas to secrete more insulin. Over time, cells that are bathed in high levels of insulin will become resistant to it, which makes it harder for your muscle, fat, and liver cells to take in the insulin. The pancreas makes more and more insulin to keep up with the increased demand, in a vicious cycle of ever-increasing insulin and insulin resistance. Eventually the overworked pancreas cannot produce enough insulin to keep the blood sugar under control. The patient has now developed type-2, or adult-onset, diabetes, a condition with persistently elevated blood sugar that is devastating to the body and the person's health.

Specific genes make people more likely to develop insulin resistance and diabetes, but a diet high in processed carbohydrates and sugar, excess weight around the middle, and a lack of physical activity definitely contribute to the problem. It's important for a woman with endo (and the rest of us!) to eat fresh, unprocessed foods to decrease the chances of developing insulin resistance, as well as to improve her overall health. A couple of years ago, when I went to the World Congress on Insulin Resistance, in San Francisco. I was impressed by all the research presented. It seems that insulin is involved in nearly every organ system in the body, from the brain (insulin may be involved in Alzheimer's disease) to the bowel.

Vitamin D

I have been checking vitamin D levels in patients for the last five years and often find low levels. It turns out vitamin D isn't really even a vitamin but an important hormone that plays many key roles, including helping to protect against cancer and autoimmune diseases, helping with insulin function, and increasing bone and muscle strength. An ever-increasing body of scientific evidence supports the importance of checking vitamin D levels and taking supplements to normalize blood levels.[64] Studies show that low vitamin D levels correlate with chronic disease.

Nearly 50,000 studies have been done on vitamin D. Numerous surveys suggest that suboptimal levels of vitamin D are widely prevalent. That may be due to a combination of factors. If you live in northern latitudes, are homebound, or have a job that limits your sun exposure, you may not get adequate sun to produce the vitamin D you need. Likewise, if you have liver disease, Crohn's disease, or cystic fibrosis, you may have problems synthesizing enough of the vitamin. If, when outside, you cover your skin and use sunscreen, you may be at greater risk of deficiency. Alcohol interferes with enzymes that help

---

64 Kennel KA, Drake MT, Hurley DL. Vitamin D deficiency in adults: when to test and how to treat. *Mayo Clinic Proceedings.* 2010;85(8):752-758.

convert vitamin D to its active form. If you are African American, you may produce only about half the vitamin D that a lighter-pigmented individual will. Also overlooked may be the role of the increasing incidence of obesity in the United States. As body-fat mass increases, vitamin D is increasingly stored in fat; the vitamin's bioavailability decreases, and its release into the circulation may be hampered.

Thyroid and Adrenal Glands

Fatigue is a common symptom of endometriosis. Depending on the patient's symptoms, it may be important to check the thyroid and/or adrenal hormone levels. There are several ways to check these hormone levels and several ways to treat them, if necessary.

The adrenal glands sit on top of the kidneys and produce many hormones that are essential for living. The adrenal gland is part of what is known as the Hypothalamic-Pituitary-Adrenal, or HPA, Axis. The hypothalamus is the part of the brain that controls the pituitary gland. The pituitary gland controls the ovaries, thyroid, and adrenal glands. In response to a stressful event, the adrenal glands release the extra stress hormones required for us to survive. Adrenal hormones include norepinephrine (adrenaline) and cortisol, among many others. Cortisol is known as the stress hormone. It can have a profound effect on the immune system, insulin function, and blood pressure; we will literally die if our cortisol levels get too low.

Traditional Western medicine and integrative healthcare practitioners differ in their opinion as to what happens with chronic long-term stress. Traditional doctors feel the adrenal gland either works or it doesn't (Addison's disease). Integrative doctors believe in adrenal fatigue, when, under chronic stress, the adrenal gland loses its ability to produce as much stress hormone as we need for optimal health. This low-level adrenal function is one of the causes of chronic fatigue. Adrenal function can be tested by blood, saliva, and urine tests. Treatment of low adrenal function can consist of either supporting the adrenal gland with the precursors needed for hormone production or simply giving small doses of hormone. Prescribing Cortef, a low-dose cortisol, for example, can normalize the cortisol deficiency.

The thyroid gland is a small gland located at the base of the neck. The gland produces thyroid hormone, which is responsible for controlling the metabolism of every cell in our bodies. It helps convert oxygen and calories into energy. Patients with endometriosis are known to have a higher incidence of hypothyroidism, or low thyroid, which can be diagnosed by checking the TSH (thyroid-stimulating hormone) level. TSH stimulates the thyroid to release the thyroid hormones T3 and T4. When the thyroid is not producing enough T3 and T4, the TSH level actually increases, to increase the output of these two hormones.

Various medical societies have differing guidelines and protocols as to which lab values constitute hypothyroidism, when thyroid replacement should be started, and even what type of thyroid hormone should be used when treating patients. Accordingly, approaches to treating hypothyroidism are similarly diverse among physicians. Many patients fall into a category known as subclinical hypothyroidism. This condition is associated with depression, memory and cognitive impairment, raised serum levels of total and LDL cholesterol, and an increased risk for the development of atherosclerosis.[65] Unfortunately, the fatigue experienced by so many patients is not often corrected with thyroid replacement.

There's still a great deal of research to be done on how all these factors affect endometriosis. But we can improve the underlying conditions by encouraging patients to be as healthy as possible: by eating properly, exercising, making sure they get enough vitamin D and other nutrients, and doing what they can to reduce stress and get a good night's sleep. All these things contribute to overall health; good health will help you heal from endometriosis.

---

65 McDermott MT, Ridgway EC. Subclinical hypothyroidism is mild thyroid failure and should be treated. *Journal of Clinical Endocrinology and Metabolism.* 2001;86(10):4585-4590.

PART III

Putting it All Together

CHAPTER NINE

The Whole Patient: Supportive and Complementary Therapies

After the endometriosis is removed by surgery, the patient may need a variety of supportive measures, depending on the individual, whether it's devising a healthy nutrition plan or relieving pain and stress. I approach helping a patient with endo, pelvic pain, and underlying and co-conditions as a team effort, with various other practitioners and therapies, including massage, acupuncture, physical therapy, psychological therapy for pain, and mind-body practices. None of these supporting therapies takes the place of surgery, but all of them can help the healing process along. Not every therapy is right for every patient; you know your body and what suits you best.

Meditation and Mindfulness

Meditation has had positive effects on the levels of pain people experience—that's how much our minds influence our bodies. How does it work? When you meditate, you concentrate on your breathing. When stray thoughts or sensations of pain arise, you notice them, note how they make you feel, and let them go. You eventually develop more mastery over how much those thoughts and feelings intrude on your life.

Researchers have found several ways of quieting the mind and eliciting the "relaxation response," including deep breathing, meditation, visualization, yoga, repetitive prayer, and mindfulness (deliberately focusing on the sensations of a small activity, like washing your hands or drinking a cup of tea). What's important is to set aside at least 15 minutes a day to sit quietly and engage in one of these activities. I've recommended Jon Kabat-Zinn's book *Full Catastrophe Living*, and I recommend his tapes as well. Many other meditation tapes, and workshops are available, but I suggest starting with Kabat-Zinn because, as director of the Stress Reduction Clinic at the University of Massachusetts Medical School, he developed his mindfulness-based stress-reduction technique mainly for people who were dealing with chronic medical conditions.[66]

Many different methods and types of activities promote mindfulness, so you should be able to find one that you can relate to and follow. Having said this, most people will find it a challenge to have the discipline to follow through on the time commitment really needed to fully implement these practices in their lives. It's a challenge, but an extremely rewarding one.

For instance, Kabat-Zinn reported that the majority of patients with chronic pain who went through the mindfulness-based stress-reduction program experienced significant reductions in their pain levels during the eight weeks they were practicing meditation. They showed a 30 percent improvement in the degree to which pain interfered with their day-to-day functioning: cooking, driving, working, sleeping, having sex. They had a 55 percent drop in negative mood states, an increase in positive mood states, and less anxiety, depression, and hostility. In general, they were much more active and felt better all around.[67]

With a chronic disease, if you can accept the pain, it is apt to lessen. "To a degree, it's not stress per se but how you are in relationship to it that makes the difference in the effects it's going to have on the mind and body," says Kabat-Zinn. "That's the area where there is a huge potential for growth, change, and hope."[68]

---

66 Jon Kabat-Zinn's meditation tapes can be found at http://www.mindfulnesscds.com

67 Kabat-Zinn J. *Full Catastrophe Living: Using the Wisdom of Your Body and Mind to Face Stress, Pain, and Illness.* 15th ed. New York, NY: Bantam Dell; 1990:288-289.

68 Jon Kabat-Zinn, interview with journalist Laura Fraser for *More* magazine, March 2005.

A recent study found that people who meditate regularly find chronic pain less unpleasant because they spend less time anticipating it. Instead, they feel it moment to moment, without catastrophizing it or helplessly thinking they will be in pain forever. In a 2010 study, researchers at the University of Manchester, England, induced pain in their subjects with a laser device. Some of the subjects had meditated for years; some did not meditate at all. The researchers found that the meditators had more activity in the prefrontal cortex, a region of the brain involved in controlling attention and thought processes when potential threats are perceived. The people who had meditated longest had the least anticipation of pain. The lead researcher, Dr. Christopher Brown, said, "Meditation trains the brain to be more present focused, and therefore to spend less time anticipating future negative events. This may be why meditation is effective at reducing the recurrence of depression, which makes chronic pain considerably worse."[69]

Another study, too, showed that mind-body medicine actually changes our brain activity (its physiology), just as physical exercise changes our muscles.[70] Dr. Magdalena Naylor, a psychiatrist and the lead investigator in a scientific study presented at the September 2010 World Congress on Pain, relates, "This shows how mind and body can work in unison and one can influence the other." Functional MRI showed activity of specific brain centers to be different in women with a history of chronic pain. This difference from "normal brains" disappeared after cognitive-behavior therapy (a type of mind-body therapy). The patients reported better coping and decreased pain. Depression, as determined by a standardized test, also decreased following mind-body therapy. A previous study showed a decrease in narcotic use, with reduced pain symptoms.[71]

---

69 Brown CA, Jones AK. Meditation experience predicts less negative appraisal of pain: electrophysiological evidence for the involvement of anticipatory neural responses. *Pain*. 2010;150(3):428-438.

70 Naylor MR, Krauthamer MG, Kumas J, Newhouse P. Treatment response to cognitive-behavioral therapy in patients with chronic pain. *13th World Congress on Pain*. Montreal, Quebec, Canada. 2010.

71 Naylor MR, Naud S, Keefe FJ, Helzer JE. Therapeutic interactive voice response (TIVR) to reduce analgesic medication use for chronic pain management. *Journal of Pain*. 2010;11(12):1410-1419.

Perhaps the most common form of meditation is sitting comfortably, closing your eyes, and following your breath. Set a timer for 15 or 20 minutes, and simply concentrate on your breath as it makes its way down into your chest and abdomen when you inhale slowly, and how it flows through your nostrils as you exhale slowly. When other thoughts arise—as they will—notice them, let go of them, and focus on your breathing again.

If you find yourself thinking, "There is no way I can do this; maybe it's for other people, but not for me," that is a big red flag. You might need "it" even more than those "other people." A triathlete finds it easy, even pleasurable, to exercise; out-of-shape people have great difficulty getting started. Similarly, a mind that is "out of shape" from living with chronic pain needs the consistent exercise and conditioning of mind-body practices. Just as with physical exercise, start slowly, even if it's just five minutes a day, and work up to longer stretches of time. You can do it! But first you have to start. Why not today?

❊ ❊ ❊

"I find that when I meditate on a regular basis, I can manage much better than when I don't. Before, I felt like the pain was running my life, like my life was over. Mindfulness helps you not to think about the past or worry about the future. If I can ask myself, 'Can I manage this pain right in this moment?' the answer is usually yes. If it's not, I can work with my limits, instead of being angry and upset and frustrated. Those things create more tension in my body, and more pain. Meditation opened up new ways of being. I'm stronger and more flexible than I was. Before, I felt I had to be a supermom, carry on no matter how bad I was feeling, and just suffer. Now, if I need to cry or take a bath, that's okay. Knowing that I can be kinder and more compassionate to myself, that there are things I need to do to be okay, makes it easier." —Connie

Pain Psychology and Counseling

As if constant physical pain wasn't enough to deal with, endometriosis can create a great deal of emotional pain, including depression. This isn't a weakness but a natural response to very difficult physiological changes. While most people would benefit from seeing a therapist, the added stress of chronic pain makes it even more important to take care of yourself. I often recommend that my patients see a therapist, ideally a psychologist who specializes in the issues associated with chronic pain.

When you have pain, your nervous system is altered. The autonomic nervous system—the one that controls many bodily functions below our consciousness (blood pressure, bowel function, etc)—has two branches. The sympathetic nervous system is about reaction, arousal, stimulation, and excitation: it revs us up ("fight or flight"). The parasympathetic nervous system calms us down and helps us regroup. (I affectionately call this the Jimmy Buffet center.) In our stressful culture, we all have overstimulated sympathetic nervous systems. Chronic pain constantly stimulates the sympathetic nervous system, causing a dominance and imbalance over the natural calming effect of the parasympathetic nervous system.

As a result, in addition to the chronic pain, people are often stressed, depressed, and tired all the time, with difficulty sleeping. The body feels like it's on the front lines, constantly reacting to stimulation, overwhelmed. My friend and colleague Douglas Drucker, PhD, a pain psychologist, says, "It's like battle fatigue or Post-Traumatic Stress Disorder. People are worn out."

Social problems contribute to the psychological stress of chronic pain. As Drucker points out, everyone is waiting for you to heal and get better. But this is a long, enduring illness. After a while, the people around you may begin to assume that you're just exaggerating or feigning illness. "A lot of estrangement and isolation occurs with endo," says Drucker. "People are sad, they're lonely, and they're pulling away from the very things that could help them."

Endometriosis can wreak havoc on relationships and marriages. It isn't easy to be with someone who is in constant pain, with low energy and depressed. That can lead to feelings of resentment, of guilt or frustration at not being able to help her, as well as a sense of loss, for the relationship you used to have and the things you used to do. Most couples could benefit from some counseling.

On top of that is the sense that you can't even count on yourself. "Your body becomes your betrayer," says Drucker. That resonates deeply with anyone; if you can't trust your body, you can't trust yourself. "There's a tearing apart of an essential relationship to the self, which is as destructive as anything, a real loss of who you are."

These are all devastating issues, but they also offer an opportunity to make a fundamental shift in how you're dealing with your pain and your life. People need to learn to have realistic expectations. We think of our bodies as machines, and when they break down, we feel betrayed; we think everything is falling apart. That's not really the case. People are very resilient. For people in pain, the resilience needs to be about accepting what they've got and moving forward.

Being in chronic pain is like aging. Eventually we will all have to deal with a loss of functioning. Older people know they can't lift that hundred-pound sack, so they don't try; they get someone else to do the heavy lifting. Accepting that things have changed, recognizing limitations, and feeling okay about it is surely a better way to live.

Resiliency is saying, "I don't have to like what's going on, but I can accept it and move on with it." That's emotional maturity, something one can strive for, learn, and adopt. Drucker says, "It's like the difference between an adult and a little kid. A kid will pitch a fit if he gets strawberry ice cream instead of chocolate. An adult will say, 'You've only got strawberry? Let me give it a try.' That's resiliency. You get what you get, and you don't have a fit." It is your choice as to how you react internally to what life presents you.

Certainly you want to do whatever you can to prevent pain and get well, and the medical changes can be miraculous. The bigger shift, though, comes when people are more accepting of whatever their body is going through.

In addition to finding a doctor who will listen to you and give you appropriate treatment, you want to get as much emotional support as you can. Support groups are a great place to start, because people with similar symptoms will understand you and ease your sense of isolation. Speaking with a counselor or psychologist can help you cope. Mind-body therapies, such as meditation and visualization, can literally rebalance your brain physiology, helping the stress centers take a break and toning up the calming parasympathetic nervous system. These therapies can be very helpful in dealing with the emotional challenges of endometriosis.

Pelvic-floor Physical Therapy

Women with endometriosis often have a condition called pelvic-floor dysfunction, when pain has caused the muscles in the pelvis to become too tight. In severe cases, they have pelvic-floor spasm, which is excruciatingly painful, making intercourse impossible. Pelvic-floor dysfunction can affect all the organs in the pelvis, as well as the urinary, genital, and bowel systems.

I refer many of my patients to a very specialized physical therapist, who treats pelvic-floor dysfunction and pelvic pain. Most physical therapists do not have training in specifically treating pelvis pain or pelvic-floor spasm. You'll need a referral from your doctor to a physical therapist with those skills.

Pelvic-floor physical therapy helps a patient stop perpetuating habits her body has developed because of the pain she's been in. The whole body can become tense and clenched from the pain radiating from the pelvis. If, for instance, a patient often lies on her side in the fetal position, she will need to learn how to relax and lengthen those muscles. Indeed, the pain in her pelvis can affect how she moves and walks, causing changes in alignment and functioning of bones and muscles from the head to the feet. Since the pain can affect the structure of the entire body, the physical therapist helps a patient realign and balance her body.

Denise Alberto, who works near me in Los Gatos and specializes in this type of physical therapy, treats many patients with endometriosis and pelvic pain. One of the things I admire about her is her willingness to listen to the patient's story. "The patient has usually been put off by the medical profession," she says. "I want to connect with her body's story, from beginning to end, so that she feels like a whole person." Alberto asks not only for the patient's history of endometriosis and attempts at treatment but about anything that might have jostled the pelvis, such as a fall while skiing or riding a horse.

Then she does extensive biomechanical and musculoskeletal evaluations: getting a sense of how the patient moves, where she hurts, and how strong, contracted, and coordinated her muscles are. She'll notice whether the patient has an imbalance in her walking because she isn't integrating her pelvic floor or is using it too much.

She even considers the patient's breathing. With proper inhalation, breath goes deep into the body, lowering the diaphragm and the pelvic floor. Many women who have been in pelvic pain do not breathe deeply, using the muscles higher in the chest and neck. Learning to breathe properly can help organ and muscle mobility and bring oxygen to the muscles and tissues, which helps in pain relief.

After that, she teaches the patient to relax as she massages her and shows her how to massage herself, to relieve pelvic and abdominal pain and mobilize the muscles in those areas. "A lot of women who have been in pain freeze when they're touched," says Alberto. "We teach you how to give yourself some healing energy through your own hands."

Then she does a thorough physical exam. She finds out, for instance, if the patient has high arches or if her arches have collapsed, and how that affects how she moves. She sees if the woman's feet are cramped up; that can influence cramping in the pelvic-floor muscle. She tests overall body flexibility and mobility, particularly in the hips; any joint malformation there will cause the pelvic-floor muscles to operate differently. She looks for abdominal scars, because that might indicate adhesions that reach deep into the pelvis, and she'll check the subtle mobility of the organs inside the pelvis.

As I mentioned earlier, a pelvic physical therapist does a careful internal exam, using a finger inserted in the vagina to check the layers of the pelvic floor. She'll feel how relaxed or contracted the muscles are, how mobile or rigid the tissues are. Some patients are initially uncomfortable with this. But palpating the tissues is the best way to evaluate the pelvic-floor muscles and other structures for mobility and restrictions and where the pain is triggered.

The therapist teaches a patient to relax, or "down train," pelvic muscles that have been clenched or are in spasm. The muscles have been in spasm and pain for so long that the patient cannot feel relaxation or contraction in the muscle. The therapist may place biofeedback sensors on the muscles; the patient can see on the biofeedback monitor the muscle activity in the pelvic floor and use this information to learn to relax or activate those muscles.

She usually gives the patient some stretching exercises to open the hips and lengthen the associated muscles. She'll give her vaginal-dilation exercises to do with a finger or a home-dilation kit (which consists of several graduated cylinders with a handle) to mobilize the tissue in the pelvis. She'll go through exercises to help trunk and spine flexibility and core strength and stability. Once pain levels are reduced and mobility is improved, she'll retrain the patient to stand, walk, and move in ways that will not make the pelvic floor contract too much. She will help the patient improve her overall pelvic-girdle coordination as well.

Walking is literally the first step. Starting with daily walks on level surfaces, the patient will progress to varied surfaces at a faster pace. Alberto recommends gentle, "restorative" yoga—not athletic power yoga—as well as Pilates mat classes, which are gentle ways to increase core strength while breathing correctly and being aware of the pelvic floor. She recommends mild exercise even during menstrual pain: "Movement helps; freezing doesn't." By the end of 6 to 12 weekly or biweekly visits, the patient should feel her pain lessened and her mobility improved.

Nutrition

Nutrition is the cornerstone of good health. It's true that you are what you eat: what you put into your body affects how it functions. For women with endometriosis, good nutrition can reduce symptoms and pain and provide a feeling of vital force in your life. Eating well can give you energy, balance your blood-sugar levels, fight insulin resistance, regulate your bowels, help balance your metabolism, and control your weight. The basis of a good diet is simple: avoid processed food with its long lists of sometimes unintelligible ingredients, and eat real, recognizable, whole foods. Processed, dead food depletes you of energy. Fresh food, with plenty of vegetables, helps you feel vital.

I screen my patients for vitamin D deficiencies and to get an idea of what they're eating, but I usually refer them to the Vital Health nutritionist. A nutritionist can help you understand which foods can increase inflammation and the production of prostaglandins and which foods can have a beneficial effect on your system.

One of the first things that Lene Joy, a nutritionist at Vital Health Institute, does is to determine whether any symptoms or pain are caused by food sensitivities. The two biggest culprits here are wheat and dairy, both of which can promote inflammation. Generally she has a patient start by eliminating foods in both categories for two weeks. It may be challenging to change old habits, but if it works, you'll be living with a lot less pain.

"After a couple of weeks, I see how the patient feels," Joy explains. "If she feels good, we'll try putting wheat back into her diet and see how she reacts." I believe that dairy products are not very healthy for any of us: dairy is a primary food source of dioxins. But milk products can be particularly harmful for women with endometriosis. A single glass of milk exposes a woman to 59 growth factors and hormones intended for a different species.[72] Joy also recommends taking food-allergy tests, to find other foods that may be causing problems. Once she has the information she needs, she works with each patient to create a reasonable food plan.

Just changing the way you eat can have a remarkable effect on how you feel. Depending on the patient, foods that increase inflammation or promote the production of pain-producing prostaglandins are sugar, alcohol, wheat, red meats, and saturated fats. If a glass of wine or a piece of chocolate makes you feel better, you might want to indulge a little. How much you should eat of a beneficial or inflammatory food is a good topic to take up with your nutritionist.

Joy recommends concentrating on seasonal and organic foods. She recommends that patients eat all vegetables (other than nightshades, which include bell peppers, potatoes, tomatoes, and eggplant), whole grains (excluding wheat, if indicated), and walnut and olive oils. For protein, she recommends fish, lots of raw nuts and legumes, and small amounts of white meats, such as chicken and veal. Since every cell requires a building block of protein, she likes her patients to eat some protein—which the body uses to repair and heal itself—with every meal. Overall, the diet she recommends is what we call the Mediterranean diet, with or without wheat, depending on the patient.

Joy's diet recommendations are different for each woman. But in general, here are some things to eat if you have endo:

- *Foods with omega-3 fatty acids* Prostaglandins come from fatty acids. "Good" prostaglandins are soothing; "bad" ones can increase uterine contractions and inflammation. The best fats contain omega-3 fatty acids. Good sources include salmon, flax seed, and walnuts, also fish-oil supplements (see below).

- *Foods with phytoestrogens* Phytoestrogens, weak hormones found in many plants, seem to block estrogen receptors, keeping excess estrogen from attaching to the

---

72 Keon J, *Whitewash, The Disturbing Truth About Cows Milk and Your Health.* New Society Publishers. 2010:103

receptors. Foods that contain phytoestrogens include apples, flax seed, hummus, garlic, green beans, dried dates, dried prunes, peaches, strawberries, raspberries, nuts and seeds, brassicas (such as cauliflower and cabbage), fennel, parsley, sage, rosemary, and thyme.

- *High-fiber foods* Fiber helps with digestion and bowel health; it may also decrease the estrogen circulating in your body. Good sources of fiber are legumes, whole grains (except wheat, for some), oatmeal, and most fruits and vegetables.

- *Foods that help with estrogen metabolism* In the previous chapter, I mentioned that certain vegetables can help estrogen metabolize in a healthy way. These include broccoli, Brussels sprouts, arugula, chard, mustard greens, turnips, kale, bok choy, radishes, and watercress.

- *Foods that are good for the immune system* Various studies have shown that certain foods have beneficial effects on the immune system. These foods include garlic, ginger, onions, carrots, legumes, rhubarb, seeds, live yogurt, and green tea.

Naturopathic Medicine

Naturopathic doctors are exposed to Western medicine in their training, but their approach comes from a philosophy that the body is capable of healing itself. They focus on supporting that process and finding obstacles to healing. It is a holistic approach, taking mind, body, and spirit into consideration, as well as diet, stress management, exercise, and sleep. They often prescribe herbal and homeopathic remedies, massage, acupuncture, and other holistic treatments to optimize a patient's health.

As with all healthcare approaches relevant to my patients, I want to make sure the naturopathic care is coordinated with my treatment. Things can get confusing and counterproductive if patients take a wide range of herbs, remedies, and supplements without coordinating it with their doctors. Also, herbs have real effects on the body, and those effects have to be balanced with the effects of the medication the patient is taking.

Dr. Amy Day is a naturopathic doctor in San Francisco. I felt she would be a great person to explain this approach, which can be an excellent complement to medical treatment and surgery—though not a replacement—because she has had surgery for endometriosis. "I'm a woman with endo, as well as a doc who treats endo," she says. "It helps my patients to have a relationship with someone who understands what's going on."

Dr. Day says stress management is crucial in dealing with chronic pain. Indeed, she feels that "the more stress you have, the more pain." She tries to mediate inflammation through diet, nutrition, and herbal approaches. She finds out if the digestive and elimination systems are functioning well. She runs month-long salivary tests, mapping out hormone levels to make sure the hormones are in balance. She may prescribe herbs, bodywork, acupuncture, homeopathy, or other complementary therapies to improve a patient's overall health.

Herbs and Supplements

Naturopaths prescribe herbs that some patients can take in lieu of painkillers. "In some cases, it's not uncommon for herbs to work better than painkillers," Dr. Day says. Patients have to be careful combining such herbs with medications prescribed by other doctors, though, and should do so only under a doctor's care.

Naturopaths individualize the supplements they prescribe. Here are some they suggest for endometriosis:

Fish oil Fish oil is high in omega-3 fatty acids, which increase anti-inflammatory prostaglandins, and has achieved good results with endometriosis.

Calcium/magnesium Magnesium, in particular, has properties that help endo patients reduce tension.

Vitamin B complex When you're under stress, you burn through your B vitamins. They give you more energy, help you deal with stress, and are necessary for producing energy in the body. Correction of

B-vitamin deficiencies, then, can help reduce stress. B-complex supplements may be beneficial, although too high a dose can cause problems as well. As with many things, moderation is good.

Herbal Pycnogenol This is pine-bark extract, an anti-inflammatory that increases blood flow. A 2007 study at the Kanazawa University School of Medicine, in Ishikawa Prefecture, Japan, showed that taking 60 mg orally of Pycnogenol (pronounced Pick-nah-geh-nol) a day reduced pain symptoms in endometriosis patients by 33 percent, and the pain relief lasted longer than with Lupron and without the drug's side effects.[73]

Diindolylmethane (DIM) Estrogen is eliminated from the body through one of three possible enzymatic reactions. One route is associated with healthy estrogen intermediates, and the other two seem to be related to a variety of diseases. DIM helps to metabolize estrogen down the good enzymatic pathway. This substance is found in cruciferous vegetables, which include broccoli, Brussels sprouts, cabbage, cauliflower, and kale. DIM can also be taken as a supplement, with daily doses of 75 mg to 300 mg. DIM can have the side effect of inhibiting thyroid function. Thus it is important to monitor patients with low thyroid function or symptoms of low thyroid function, especially when using DIM in higher doses.

Progesteronic herbs Several kinds of progesteronic herbs—herbs that have progesterone activity—help to inhibit estrogen. Suppressing estrogen activity by increasing progesterone levels is one type of treatment for endometriosis. (More information on this approach is found in chapter six.)

Vitamin D Among its other increasingly well-known benefits, vitamin D helps mediate the immune system. (See chapter eight for a more detailed discussion.)

---

73 Kohama T, Herai K, Inoue M. Effect of French maritime pine bark extract on endometriosis as compared with leuprorelin acetate. *Journal of Reproductive Medicine.* 2007;52(8):703-708.

Low-dose Naltrexone (LDN) Therapy

Naltrexone is a narcotic blocker originally synthesized in 1963 and approved by the FDA in 1984. In normal prescription doses of 50 mg, it is used to treat narcotic overdose or addiction. Low-dose Naltrexone (LDN) therapy uses very small doses, usually 3 to 4.5 mg. A pharmacist has to compound or make pills with such a small dose, as it is not available from the manufacturer in a pill of less than 50 mg.

This is probably the closest we have to an immune-enhancing pill. LDN is taken once a day, just before going to bed. The low dose acts to block our natural endorphins (the hormones behind the "runner's high") for a short period of time. The body reacts to this temporary decrease by producing more endorphins, which seems to stimulate the immune system.[74, 75] Naltrexone has been found to reduce the production of proinflammatory cytokines via suppressive effects on central nervous system microglia cells.[76]

A 2009 Stanford study using LDN to treat fibromyalgia patients showed a 30 percent decrease in symptoms.[77] The patients with the highest inflammation in this study responded the best. Eighty-nine percent of patients with Crohn's disease responded to LDN therapy; 67 percent went into remission with LDN therapy.[78] Theoretically, this therapy could benefit endometriosis patients, too. However, no studies show that LDN is effective in treating the pain of endometriosis, nor in decreasing the recurrence rate as a result of improved immune function.

---

74 Ballantyne JC, Mao J. Opioid Therapy for Chronic Pain. *New England Journal of Medicine*. 2003; 349(20):1943-1953.

75 Bidlack JM. Detection and function of opioid receptors on cells from the immune system. *Clinical and Diagnostic Laboratory Immunology*. 2000;7(5):719-723.

76 Liu B, Hong JS. Neuroprotective effect of naloxone in inflammation-mediated dopaminergic neurodegeneration: Dissociation from the involvement of opioid receptors. *Methods in Molecular Medicine*. 2002;79:43-54.

77 Younger J, Mackey S. Fibromyalgia symptoms are reduced by low-dose naltrexone: a pilot study. *Pain Medicine*. 2009;10(4):663-672.

78 Smith JP, Stock H, Bingaman S, Mauger D, Rogosnitzky M, Zagon IS. Low-dose naltrexone therapy improves active Crohn's disease. *American Journal of Gastroenterology*. 2007;102:820-828.

Bodywork

Hands-on therapeutic bodywork can relax pelvic and abdominal muscles clenched with endometriosis, as well as release stored energy. Bodywork can include such techniques as yoga, reiki, tai chi, qi gong, rolfing, shiatsu, reflexology, and chiropractic care. Individual patient needs and preferences will dictate which of these treatment modalities is best. As with any treatment, patients should be well informed about the proposed treatment, and the benefit should outweigh any side effects.

Acupuncture

Acupuncture involves placing very thin needles in various strategic places in the body. It has been practiced in China for thousands of years, and it is based on the belief that *chi*, or energy flow, through pathways (meridians) in your body can become blocked or imbalanced, resulting in disease and pain. Placing the needles at specific points along the meridian helps to rebalance this flow. A Western-medicine theory is that it may help regulate the nervous system and release pain-suppressing endorphins.

Scientific evidence indicates that acupuncture may be beneficial in helping reduce the pain associated with endometriosis.[79] Several of my patients have reported that acupuncture has offered them significant pain relief. Acupuncture also can have positive effects on the menstrual cycle, helping a woman to have a milder, less painful flow.

Homeopathy

Homeopathic medicine was developed in Germany more than 200 years ago. The idea is that a small amount of a substance that causes symptoms of a disease can help cure it, if used in minute amounts and shaken with water. It is felt that this "potentization" of the solution has energetic effects on the body. The National Center for Complementary and Alternative Medicine states that homeopathy

79   Rubi-Klein K, Kucera-Sliutz E, Nissel H, Bijak M, Stockenhuber D, Fink M, Wolkenstein E. Is acupuncture in addition to conventional medicine effective as pain treatment for endometriosis? A randomized controlled cross-over trial. *European Journal of Obstetrics and Gynecology Reproductive Biology*. 2010;153(1):90-93.

is a controversial area of integrative medicine, because a number of its key concepts are not consistent with the laws of chemistry and physics. Regardless, it is estimated that 3.3 million adults spent nearly $3 billion purchasing homeopathic medicine in 2007.[80] It is unlikely that homeopathic remedies will cause any harm. The question is if it will help the patient's condition.

Craniosacral Therapy

The craniosacral system includes the membranes and fluid that surround the brain and spinal cord. The bones of the skull and spinal column are part of the craniosacral system extending from the skull down into the pelvic area. Over time, trauma and biomechanical changes can limit cranial-bone movement and distort the flow of CSF fluid. Craniosacral therapy is a gentle therapy that practitioners say eases restrictions in the nerve passages in the spine and facilitates movement of the cerebrospinal fluid through the spinal cord.[81] They use the therapy for chronic pain, neck pain, back pain, as well as for mental stress. It seems to offer significant relief to some endometriosis and pelvic-pain patients, but not others. It probably depends on whether the patient has a condition that can be helped by this type of therapy.

✿ ✿ ✿

"I've sought out every option I can in dealing with pain: herbal remedies, meditation, exercise, diet, mind concentration. I've tried every avenue, and I have to say that to be a functioning adult, I pretty much rely on ibuprofen and mind-over-matter coping skills. I call it going Zen. You try not to focus on your pain; you focus on other things. Otherwise, your quality of life is going to be very poor.

---

80 Nahin RL, Barnes PM, Stussman BJ, Bloom B. Costs of Complementary and Alternative Medicine (CAM) and Frequency of Visits to CAM Practitioners:United States, 2007. U.S. Department Of Health And Human Services. *National Health Statistics Reports.* July 30, 2009. Number 18. http://www.cdc.gov/nchs/data/nhsr/nhsr018.pdf

81 Biodynamic Craniosacral Therapy Association of North American. http://www.craniosacraltherapy.org. Accessed June 12, 2011.

"The average person doesn't even know how to say endometriosis, let alone understand what it is. I got into a real tussle with my friends. I told them, 'Look, if you want to pass judgment on me, you'd better be ready to explain the illness, and then we'll talk.' A pain counselor explained that boundaries are the key with endo. If you're working with a crowd that doesn't understand it, you've just got to say, 'No, thanks, I've got other plans.'" —Kathleen

"Once I found a doctor who explained what was going on, I felt better. But you get so used to not feeling well that it affects how you interact with people. I remember coming out on the other side of all of this thinking, 'Boy, that really took a toll on everything.'" —Kaela

After reading about all these alternative therapies, you may wonder where you'll find time to do anything but go to acupuncture and massage appointments, meditate, chop vegetables, and take supplements. The list of complementary health options can seem overwhelming. Not all of them will be appropriate for you or your budget. I want to help you adopt a positive lifestyle, which will support optimal health, by building a strong foundation for proper functioning. Hopefully you will have a team of practitioners who can work together and support you. But ultimately, you're the one in charge of your health, and you'll know which of these therapies is helping you.

CHAPTER TEN

Back to Vital Health

I view every patient as a collaborator in her health. Her lifestyle choices and frame of mind can make a huge difference in her recovery. My staff and I provide our skills, knowledge, and expertise not only to help her get rid of endometriosis but also to support her in improving her overall physical, emotional, and even spiritual well-being.

No matter how healthy a patient's way of living is, of course, if she has endometriosis, she needs to have it removed; with proper surgery, it will be in remission and possibly never recur, meaning that the patient is effectively "cured." While removal of endometriosis is a critical first step, it's usually not the only step. The best outcomes in treating virtually any chronic disease are achieved with a multidisciplinary approach—which can include functional medicine—to treat underlying disease conditions and co-conditions. With endometriosis, this approach can be absolutely critical in achieving a successful outcome.

In my practice, we get rid of most of the pain in most of the patients and get rid of all the pain in a significant percentage of our patients, including ones who have been through multiple surgeries and have been told it is hopeless. Unfortunately, some patients have many of the co-conditions we see with this complex disease. And sometimes the pain with endometriosis or associated conditions, such as neuropathic pain, interstitial cystitis, and bladder pain, can never be completely eliminated. In those cases, the healing process entails not only minimizing physical pain but changing the woman's relationship to it.

Something I did not expect to see when I started treating patients with endo is their strength and determination. When I think of my patients, I often think of the lotus, a beautiful flower that can thrive in the dirtiest waters, bringing beauty out of the most awful circumstances. The flower represents regeneration, purity, and rebirth. Over the years, I have seen so many women take a horrible situation and turn it into an opportunity for growth and development.

Real healing comes with acceptance of the state of your body at that moment, with optimism that life can still be full. Real healing comes from changing your relationship to pain—from one filled with anger, hopelessness, anxiety, and despair to one full of gentleness, awareness, and compassion for yourself and your body.

You may be thinking that's easy for me to say. I'm a guy; I've never suffered the constant pain of endometriosis. And in many ways, you're right. But the truth is, all of us eventually have to go through difficult changes in our lives, whether it's chronic disease, divorce, accidents, the death of loved ones, or the indignities of aging. Resiliency, as my pain-psychologist friend Doug Drucker says, comes from accepting such changes.

In many ways, having a chronic disease is an opportunity to create a fundamental shift in how you look at and deal with life, including challenges you'll have to face down the road. In other words, there's another aspect to successfully treating endometriosis. My goals are to get rid of as much pain as possible and to help the woman live positively with the outcome.

Moving Back Into Normal Life

Most patients feel that if they can just be free of their pain, they can get back to living the life they once knew. Returning to a normal, functional life, however, is not as simple as most people would think. Patients, their families, and even healthcare professionals rarely understand this aspect of dealing with endometriosis and pelvic pain. Everyone, including the patient, expects that everything will be fine. But once the pain that's been front and center for so many years is greatly diminished or gone, issues that have been simmering beneath the surface become more apparent.

Just as with any relationship that's been violated, renewing your trust in your body isn't always easy. In addition to a sense of betrayal by your own body, the issues can include disappointment in friends, family members, and co-workers who didn't understand; anger at the medical system; and, mostly, a great sense of loss. For women who are suddenly pain free, it can be devastating to realize they could have spent years feeling good—instead of being in excruciating pain—if they had had the correct treatment to begin with. It's not uncommon for women to feel sad or depressed, wondering why they don't feel relieved and happy. "For a lot of women, it's the first time they've felt good enough to realize how much they've lost," Drucker explains. "It's a grieving process."

All these feelings are normal. It takes time to grieve. It takes time to realize that your body isn't going to turn on you again. Returning to a normal life after years of being nonfunctional is like getting out of jail after a long incarceration. It would seem you're free to do anything you want, but it's a big process, with several layers. Many people feel worse before they feel better, because, without pain in the foreground, they become aware of so much else in their lives.

Ideally, you will emerge from this transition being much more awake than you were before, living life more fully. It's an incredible opportunity, really. But you can't rush it. If you find yourself feeling melancholy or angry, remember: there is nothing wrong with you. It's just another part of the healing process. Consider Dr. Elisabeth Kubler-Ross's five stages of grief: denial and isolation; anger; bargaining; depression; and acceptance. This will help you recognize your feelings for what they are.

If you're not already working with a counselor, this may be a good time to start. Or, if you have a significant other, to find a relationship counselor. Better to acknowledge, accept, and deal with the challenges than to let them fester and grow. Remember the lotus flower: beauty growing out of filthy water. Your life with endo was not what you would have chosen, but it's given you a chance to reach new heights as a human being. Some of the most beautiful people are endo patients. Yes, now you are beginning to understand!

The Mind-Body Connection

While most of us have heard of "living in the moment" or the expression "be here now," few of us actually live life this way. Most of us spend most of our time in the past or the future, drawing conclusions from a past experience or conjuring possible consequences of a future event. In essence, we spend most of our lives in the past, fretting about what would have, could have, or should have been. But we can do nothing about the past or the future; we can only act on the present. What is happening in real time, right now, is the only reality.

Mind-body practice, such as meditation, keeps us from spending so much time in the fantasyland of past and future. It helps us be present in the present, which is the only place we can truly live. Once you grasp this concept, a whole new world will open up to you—one that is genuinely remarkable, no matter what your current situation is.

Meditation, says Jon Kabat-Zinn, involves accepting things as they are, without judgment. "Acceptance doesn't mean passive resignation. If you can accept the moment you are in now, whether it is painful or joyful, understanding that it is the fullest moment you have, your anxieties about pain or the future diminish. Meditation is really about reclaiming your life as if it were worth living now," he says.[82]

I wrote about Kabat-Zinn's program at the Stress Reduction Clinic at the University of Massachusetts Medical School in the previous chapter. Not only did the majority of patients in the program feel less pain while practicing meditation; they developed more self-confidence and optimism, as well as greater acceptance of themselves and their limitations.[83]

---

82 Jon Kabat-Zinn, interview with journalist Laura Fraser for *More* magazine, March 2005.

83 Kabat-Zinn J. *Full Catastrophe Living: Using the Wisdom of Your Body and Mind to Face Stress, Pain, and Illness.* 15th ed. New York, NY: Bantam Dell; 1990:38-39.

It may be hard to believe that closing your eyes and concentrating on your breathing is going to make big changes in your life. I quoted Connie, one of my patients, in that chapter. She and her husband, Jeff, have been together for 22 years. After many years, all her endometriosis has been removed, but associated conditions are still causing her pain, including neuropathic pain.

"As a male, I wanted to fix everything," says Jeff. "I thought, 'Let's knock out the disease and move on.' Then you realize it's not that easy. That's when I started tapping into meditation as well." It helped him to realize that Connie's chronic pain wasn't static. "If you think it will never change," he says, "it's catastrophic, and you feel it's running your life. It's always awful. With Connie, I've noticed that if you use pain as a sort of tool for your meditation, instead of as a giant enemy, you can learn more about yourself."

The notion of impermanence has helped the couple let go of expectations and be more flexible. "We have to deal with her pain on a daily or moment-by-moment basis," Jeff says. "Today we might not do what we said we were going to do. It just comes down to knowing that everything is changing anyway, so why can't the days change, our plans change?"

I am in awe of people like Connie and Jeff, of their positive attitudes and their willingness to accept life as it is. Even in a worst-case scenario like Connie's, it is possible to live a fulfilling life. I wish that kind of mindfulness and awareness for all my patients, because I know how much it will help them to lead fuller lives, too.

(That doesn't mean we give up on finding ways to reduce the pain. I am always looking for ways to better treat this terrible disease!)

Back to Sexual Vitality

In many areas of medicine, painful sex or decreased libido are viewed as matter-of-fact side effects of endo, not to be taken very seriously. But that's the sort of thinking that keeps people from taking endometriosis seriously—it's a "woman's problem." That's very antiquated thinking, not to mention unnecessary.

I believe positive sexual health is integral to your overall health and attitude—that healing from endometriosis often includes sexual healing. With endo, it's not unusual to reach a point where you think of your body only in relation to pain. You can't imagine experiencing any pleasure from it; that becomes a foreign concept. Even when you're better, and the idea makes sense intellectually, feeling emotionally ready for sex can be a whole other step. If you've repeatedly burned yourself on a stove, you're going to be apprehensive about touching it again, even if you know for a fact that the stove was turned off and has been cold for hours.

Some patients manage to get back to a pleasurable, exciting sexual relationship on their own—that is, with a lot of self-healing, patience, and exploration and communication with their partner. If a woman has had pain for a long time, though, it's often difficult to return to a fulfilling sex life. She can't help being wary of pain. That's when I refer people to a sexologist or sex therapist. Sex therapists tend to treat psychological disorders around sex. Sexologists tend to counsel people on any sexual issues that come up between the partners. Both can be useful, but it's always best to get a referral and interview the counselor first, to make sure you feel comfortable with him or her.

Amy Cooper PhD, a sexologist, has endometriosis, so she understands the challenges very well. Whether a couple is still dealing with painful sex or recovering after painful sex, Cooper starts by discussing their sexual bond, as well as basic issues about intimacy. She has each talk about what is going on with him or her sexually and then asks the other to reflect on what was said; to appreciate what the partner has gone through; and to note what is good and working for them. "I want to build compassion," she says. She gives some couples exercises to build intimacy, such as "hand on heart," where one person lies down, the other puts his or her hand on heart, and the person lying down shares his or her feelings.

"Each partner gets a chance to dive into what they're feeling and experiencing," Cooper notes. "This dynamic is different with every couple. Often, there's one person in the relationship with big feelings, and the other listens a lot, and the listener ends up putting his or her feelings on the back burner. It's important for both parties to have their feelings expressed and heard."

She often helps the couple deal with shame. "Usually people are unaware they have shame, but we need to deal with whatever uncomfortable feelings they have about sex. Not that we delve into childhood issues, but a lot of people have had childhoods with a lack of physical contact or nurturing and a denial of sexual feelings."

Then she helps the couple express what they like sexually. "With the woman, I ask, 'What would feel good to you? How much sexuality can you handle right now?' Maybe she just needs to cuddle and be held; maybe she'd like a massage, maybe to give a massage; and maybe she's willing to pleasure him, as a gift to him, because she has compassion for him."

Cooper often helps women understand men's sexuality. "They don't really get it," she says. "They don't believe that men's sex drives are inherently stronger than women's. They have all this testosterone, and it's a wonderful thing, but it creates a discrepancy. Men often feel judged for their sex drives, and they have a lot of guilt and shame. Women can have more compassion for men about that. It doesn't mean they have to 'give in'; it just means they have compassion, because they don't know what it's like to be sexually frustrated."

Then she helps the man have more compassion for the woman. "A man needs to learn that it's not all about his needs. He needs to learn to take care of himself in ways he can. Or learn ways that he can give to her that will make her more likely to give to him. They can pleasure each other differently: he can give her a massage; she can give him a hand job. It doesn't have to be the same thing, but you can recognize that this is what you value most."

In general, Cooper says, if you're a woman who has always enjoyed sex, it'll be easier to be intimate again: "You're going to be back on the horse a lot sooner." If you have never really enjoyed sex (perhaps because you've always had pain with sex), then it will take a little longer to figure out how to have a satisfying sex life.

For women who still have pain with intercourse, Cooper recommends the couple take their time and explore each other manually and orally. She is a big advocate of women self-pleasuring. "Play with yourself, because you're the safest person. You can adjust something instantly if it starts to hurt. If the man takes care of his needs, and she takes care of hers, they can find ways of connecting intimately through loving touch, cuddling, kissing. Gradually she can coach him on what degree of contact she's ready for, and how she would like to be touched." (We are using the example of a female and male couple, but the same advice applies to lesbian couples.)

Cooper says that endometriosis can be a chance for couples to create a new kind of intimacy. "There are so many things that can happen in people's lives that mean they can't be sexual for a while. This is an opportunity to get closer and to build your emotional bond, which will deepen your sexual bond, too."

One of my patients shared how she was able to get back to being sexual after endometriosis surgery, and found herself feeling sexier than ever:

> "Dealing with endometriosis has been one of my greatest challenges. I've had three surgeries, the last being a hysterectomy with ovaries still intact. The road to recovery has been long and painful, but I am happy now. Endometriosis causes debilitating pain, and the pain during sex was unbearable. Sex was not pleasurable; instead, I felt sharp, very intense pain with any insertion or thrusting. I would cry, because I felt like I was being kicked in the stomach. I wasn't having orgasms; my muscles were tight and clenched from years of endo.

> "After my second surgery, I found a pelvic physical therapist. She would use a glove and insert her fingers, massaging the tight areas of my pubococcygeus (pc) muscle. I did biofeedback, practicing Kegel exercises, so I could see on the monitor how much I was able to contract and relax.

This helped my brain and body re-synch. I also used a dilator (given to me by my pelvic physical therapist), which I inserted at home to help stretch my muscles. I gave myself belly and vaginal massages with oil and aromatherapy.

"I started using a vibrator, but I wasn't having orgasms. I barely felt anything—maybe because my nerves were so used to feelings of pain, I couldn't feel the subtler sensations. I was frustrated and angry, because nothing was happening! I decided to back off using the vibrator, just using it on a slow speed and for a shorter time, even though I didn't orgasm.

"Looking back, I was being very hard on myself. I was dealing with many emotions: anger, feelings of not being enough, less than a 'woman,' shame that I couldn't be with my boyfriend, and pressure to 'perform.' That's not to mention his frustration that he wasn't able to 'please me.' I was so frustrated at the state my body was in. Not only were clitoral orgasms difficult for me, but deriving pleasure from my g-spot was also stunted. Additionally, the pain of endo was depressing for me, and this also affected my sex drive. It was a vicious cycle on all levels. I had to really practice self-love and acceptance. I decided to back off and let my body go at its own pace.

"I was still having painful, heavy menstruation and some residual pain following the second surgery. Afterwards, I continued my rehabilitation, went to pelvic physical therapy a few more times, and finally my muscles normalized.

"I made 'date nights' with myself. I'd light candles, play music, used a body pillow to elevate my pelvis, and continued with the Kegels and belly rubs. I would use a hot-water compress vaginally while I used oil and fingers to self-pleasure. The heat helped me relax further. I began having orgasms again, but it only happened with a vibrator. Eventually I used a combination of vibrator and fingers; I'd self-pleasure with fingers and, once I was close to climax, used the vibrator to have an orgasm. I continued to do this regularly (practice, practice, practice), and orgasms were gradually becoming easier and more intense. Now I orgasm regularly with just fingers and have strong contractions during my orgasms. I am a year post-op and feel great. I still have to adjust my body during certain positions, most likely due to adhesions, but this is manageable. My sexuality has opened and expanded like never before." —Kelli

Advice from Patients

It's my patients who are the real experts on endometriosis. They know their bodies, and they've been wonderful collaborators in the healing process. Every day I am mindful of what incredible women I work with, how much they've gone through, and how resilient they are in the face of this very difficult, complex disease. They have refused to be defeated, and many have ended up living lives that are fuller, wiser, and more passionate because of the journey they've been through. I want to close by sharing some of the advice these incredible women have to offer.

"There are things you have to cut out of your life if you want to manage endo. I had to be on guard when I went to restaurants, because eating rich, heavy food every night exacerbated my endo. I was working in the food and wine industry, but realized to heal myself I needed to get out of that environment of rich food, drinking, and not resting. I'm in the process of going back to school and getting a new career.

"Whatever works, do it. Eat for your illness: cutting out processed foods, eating relatively vegetarian, staying away from sugars and wheat products; no alcohol, no fried foods, no smoking or drinking. I use an herbal supplement that addresses inflammation, and probiotics that help my digestion. You don't have to be bound by Western medicine.

"Learn how to be nice to yourself. Don't feel guilty that you're ill. Go into it, embrace it, and deal with it. Take care of yourself. Avoid people who don't understand your illness, including physicians." —Kathleen

"It sounds strange, but the endometriosis taught me a lot. It taught me how to fight for myself. It showed me how strong I can be. And to keep going until you find the right answer. I am thankful for my doctor, who as far as I am concerned is my savior, for my husband, and for my son. It all came together because I didn't quit." —Lillyth

"I've had a total of 11 surgeries. Through all of this, I have matured—grown emotionally and spiritually. I am so grateful for my doctor and his wonderful staff. I am thankful for my therapist, and for family and friends who listened to me cry, brought groceries when I could not shop, drove me home from the hospital, and lent me their hope when I had none of my own. Today I am 40 years old. I have completed my master's degree in social work. I am on my way to becoming a licensed therapist." —Elizabeth

"After my surgery, my pain was completely gone. What would I do with my new life? I started a chocolate company. I had taken an internship with a similar company; I watched the Food Network; I thought, 'I can do this!' It was in my blood. After all, my dad owned a Chinese restaurant in the 1970s and '80s, and I worked in the restaurant for nine years; my grandmother owned a catering business. So on Valentine's Day I launched my chocolate business. But something even bigger was happening. Before the surgery, the pain had dominated me; now I was less repressed. I became more outspoken. I felt I deserved more. Pain keeps you down—you don't just feel it; you live it. Now I was pain free, and my authentic personality came through." —I-Li

"I'm married to my best friend, and I can always count on him to be there. So many women don't have that. Being in love is certainly helpful. After that, keeping an open mind and being able to communicate and talk things out, to ask questions, discuss things. My faith helps get me where I want to be, so that's huge. Not every family has that faith, but they find ways. We meditate a lot, stay quiet and calm, and do a lot of exercises together. It's been a long journey, but you learn the red flags and green flags along the way: knowing what to be aware of, what to ask questions about." —Peggy

"I often counsel other guys about endo. Patience is the biggest thing, I tell these guys. Then there's education. I tell them to learn as much as they can about the disease, physically and mechanically, what's there, and why intercourse may be painful. Some men are willing to talk fairly openly about those things, and others are not. I just try to instill in them a sense of caring, to be involved with the disease and the healing. It comes down to loving your partner. You made a commitment for better or worse, and you just hold her up in love." —Peggy's husband, Roy

"The main thing is to trust your instincts. We fall short of that because most of us don't have the education, knowledge, or experience our doctors have. What we don't understand is that most of them don't know, either. You can end up bitter and angry at the medical profession, because what they do is hide their ignorance. They wouldn't listen: it was in my head, it was menopause, it was everything but 'they don't know.' Every little thing that we feel, experience, and deal with is part of endo. You've got to write down what you're going through, all your feelings and symptoms. I did a little bit of journaling and a lot of praying before I got to my doctor. My instincts knew I'd found the right help." —Kelli

"Endometriosis has taught me a lot. It has shown me that I must face the pain and I must care for myself. Instead of giving in to my disease, I will conquer it. I am proud of myself for not giving up. Who knows what the future will bring, but I am ready. I am strong." —Lisa

Time for a Change

The challenges in treating endometriosis and pelvic pain high-light the shortcomings in our general method of treating disease. Traditional Western medicine is primarily a disease-management system. For a complex disease such as endometriosis, the medical treatment is all too often disorganized and marginally effective—an approach that can lead to blaming the patient for her condition when she does not respond to treatment as expected. As with many chronic diseases, however, endometriosis is beyond the simple one-disease management method. The comprehensive, mul-tidisciplinary approach that provides the most effective treatment of endometriosis is a far better paradigm for regaining and maintaining good health.

Our current approach to healthcare is essentially "live hard, and fix it when it breaks." That thinking is consuming an ever-increasing amount of our resources. A huge proportion of people in the United States (and beyond) are living lives full of stress, eating food with poor nutritional value, and failing to exercise on a regular basis. Obesity and chronic disease are not only on the rise; they are reaching epidemic proportions.

We need to begin to change the way we think about health and the way we treat disease. We need to understand that modern medicine can't fix the effects of a lifetime of stress, toxins, and disregard for the body. To have a more complete understanding of how chronic diseases function, we need to look at how all these factors are interwoven. The emerging field of epigenomic medicine is helping us see the significant role that our environment—not only factors such as toxins but also diet, exercise, and emotional health—plays in our health and well-being. We can't change the DNA we are born with, but evolving science is showing us that we can change the activity of certain genes and thus our risk of disease.

An intelligent medical system would look at the entire picture of a patient's health, not just at what's not working. It would listen to the patient. It would create incentives for people to become as healthy as they can, to make their bodies as inhospitable to disease as they can—not to put blame on a patient, but to emphasize that the healthier we are, the less likely we are to develop a disease and the faster we will heal. An intelligent medical system, an intelligent approach to healing, involves the mind and spirit as well. Science is beginning to understand how interconnected our minds are with the functioning of our bodies. We can't dismiss the impact of meditation and stress relief on good health.

In other words, we need a more comprehensive approach to health and disease. The reforms to the medical system begun in 2010 will not fix the healthcare system. They will only help more people gain access to this broken system. It's time to put our resources into a much bigger picture of healing so that people such as my endometriosis patients don't have to suffer needlessly for years in order to be heard, to be treated, and finally to be healed.

There Is Hope

I hope that this book will give women with endometriosis, along with their partners, friends, and families, a renewed sense of hope and optimism that good treatments are out there, as well as lots of support to help them in the healing process.

My patients have described the frustrations they've encountered with the medical system in trying to get doctors to listen to them and to get proper treatment for endometriosis. Unfortunately, this sort of scenario is played out in the United States every day about almost every sort of disease.

While many unanswered questions remain about endometriosis, we do have good, effective treatment available right now. Unfortunately, the reality of this complex disease is that some women will continue to have varying levels of pain. But it is possible for a good number of patients with endometriosis and pelvic pain to receive treatment, to have a significant reduction or even resolution of their symptoms, and to get rid of their pain. It is possible to put the disease in remission; it is possible that it may never come back.

Trust your gut feelings. Ask questions. Few doctors really understand endo and pelvic pain. Keep looking until you find the right fit for you. Travel if you have to. Find your inner strength, and settle for nothing less than achieving your optimal health in every sense of the word. You may have been dealt some crummy cards in the game of life, but from what I have seen, women with endo are tough. They are compassionate. And some are truly the embodiment of the lotus flower—great beauty growing out of unfavorable conditions.

I hope this book will help you on this journey of recovery and life. I wish the best of luck to all of you.

RESOURCES

Dr. Andrew S. Cook and Vital Health Institute
www.vitalhealth.com
www.facebook.com/VitalHealth
www.twitter.com/VitalHealth
www.vitalhealth.com/blog

Adhesions
International Adhesions Society   www.adhesions.org

Advocates for Patients
HealthCare Advocates   www.healthcareadvocates.com
Patient Advocate Foundation   www.patientadvocate.org

Blood Sugar Insulin Resistance
National Institute of Diabetes and Digestive and Kidney Diseases
    www.diabetes.niddk.nih.gov/dm/pubs/insulinresistance

Bowel Health
General information about IBS   www.aboutibs.org
Irritable Bowel Syndrome Support Group   www.ibsgroup.org
Celiac Disease Foundation   www.celiac.org

Endometriosis
Endometriosis Association   www.endometriosisassn.org
Endometriosis Foundation of America   www.endofound.org
Endometriosis Research Center   www.endocenter.org
Endometriosis UK   www.endometriosis-uk.org
Endo Resolved   www.endo-resolved.com
EndoZone   www.endometriosiszone.org
World Endometriosis Research Foundation
    www.endometriosisfoundation.org

Food Allergies
Gluten-Free products   www.glutenfree.com
Living Without magazine   www.livingwithout.com

Functional Medicine
Institute of Functional Medicine   www.functionalmedicine.org

Hysterectomy
Hysterectomy alternatives and after-effects   www.hersfoundation.com

Infertility
American Society for Reproductive Medicine   www.asrm.org
RESOLVE   www.resolve.org

Interstitial Cystitis/Painful Bladder Syndrome
Interstitial Cystitis Association   www.ichelp.org
Interstitial Cystitis Network   www.ic-network.com

Menopause
The Hormone Foundation   www.hormone.org
The North American Menopause Society   www.menopause.org

Mind-Body Medicine
Full Catastrophe Living by Jon Kabat-Zinn   www.mindfulnesscds.com

Naturopathic Medicine
American Association of Naturopathic Physicians
   www.naturopathic.org
Amy Day ND   www.DrAmyDay.com

Pain Management
American Academy of Pain Management   www.aapainmanage.org
American Chronic Pain Association   www.theacpa.org
International Pelvic Pain Society   www.pelvicpain.org
Pain Center   www.pain.com

Pain Psychology
Douglas Drucker PhD   DougDruck@aol.com

Pelvic-Floor Muscle Physical Therapy
American Physical Therapy Association   www.apta.org
Denise Alberto PT   www.denisealberto.com

Recommended Reading List
From Vital Health Institute   www.vitalhealth.com/
   patient-physician-resources/suggested-reading.php

RX List
The Internet Drug Index   www.rxlist.com

Sexuality
American Association of Sexuality Educators, Counselors,
   and Therapists   www.aasect.org
Amy Cooper PhD   www.loveyoursexlife.com

Support Groups
Endometriosis Association   www.endometriosisassn.org
Endometriosis Research Center   www.endocenter.org

Teen Health
Btweens, E-zine for teenage girls   www.btweens.com
Museum of Menstruation and Women's Health   www.mum.org
Teen Health   www.teenshealth.org

Vaginismus
Vaginismus Awareness Network
   www.vaginismus-awareness-network.org
Vaginismus.com   www.vaginismus.com

Vulvodynia
National Vulvodynia Association   www.nva.org
The VP Foundation   www.vulvarpainfoundation.org

Women's Health
Healthy Women   www.healthywomen.org
Medline Plus   www.nlm.nih.gov/medlineplus
OB/GYN.net   www.obgyn.net
Women's Health Information   www.womenshealth.gov
Women's Health Resource   www.wdxcyber.com/mhyst.htm

Tip Sheets

The following Tip Sheets were designed to be a helpful resource for you if you might have been diagnosed with or are living with endometriosis. The information here might be useful for discussions with family members or others who are giving support to you. The Tip Sheet on finding an endo doctor is a great tool if you are faced with that critically important task of finding the right doctor for you.

Do I Have Endometriosis?

There are no blood tests or x-rays that can diagnose endometriosis. Severe cases of endometriosis, especially an ovarian endometrioma (chocolate cyst) have a characteristic appearance that is highly suggestive of endometriosis, but laparoscopy (belly button surgery) is the only way to make an actual diagnosis of endometriosis.

Symptoms

While few women with endo will have all of the following symptoms, the most common symptoms are listed below:

- Severe menstrual pain (pain around or during periods) that interferes with normal life functioning, especially if the intensity of pain and number of days in pain each month increases over time.
- Deep pain with sexual intercourse; a patient might describe it by saying, "He's hitting something sore inside me."
- Painful bowel movements
- Rectal pain or bleeding
- Pain during ovulation
- Fatigue
- Back or leg pain during menstruation
- Sharp pain during orgasm
- Infertility
- Cycles of constipation and diarrhea
- Blood in the urine
- Nausea

Internal Pelvic Exam

A physical exam (PE) can glean additional information about a patient's condition. A long list of indicators looked for during a PE, especially an internal pelvic exam, helps determine if a patient has endometriosis. A PE can also be used to find other conditions contributing to pelvic pain.

Signs of endometriosis looked for during a pelvic PE include the following:

- During a bi-manual (internal) exam, the patient's pelvic pain is reproduced with pressure on the areas where endo usually grows (including the posterior cul-de-sac, cervix, pelvic side walls, and ovaries).

- The presence of specific areas that when pressed during the internal exam re-create the deep penetration pain during sex.

- One or both ovaries are enlarged, suggesting one or more endometriomas (also called chocolate cysts).

- A "frozen pelvis," meaning all of the organs are stuck to-gether in the pelvis, is seen. (Rather than being soft and moving around, the pelvis feels like concrete.)

- Nodularity (endo implants that have grown through the vagina) is present in the vagina.

Transvaginal Ultrasound

Transvaginal ultrasound (sonogram) can be another helpful tool in diagnosing endometriosis, especially if the endometriosis surgeon does it personally, even though endo cannot usually be seen directly. Sonograms have several advantages as a diagnostic tool:

- Sonograms can be used as a type of pain mapping, applying gentle pressure with the ultrasound wand. This allows the doctor to pinpoint the location of the pain while looking at exactly what structure or area inside is causing the pain.

- Areas evaluated during sonographic pain mapping should include the posterior cul-de-sac, cervix, para-rectal spaces, uterus, both ovaries, the pelvic sidewalls, the bladder, the wall of the rectum, and the groin area.

- Scar tissue cannot be seen directly, but with gentle pres-sure in and out, all of the organs should move separately and roll over each other. If they all move together, they are likely stuck together with scar tissue.

- Occasionally endometriosis can be seen in the wall of the rectum or in the posterior cul-de-sac if the endometriosis lesion is large enough. While this does not provide an official diagnosis by itself, the possibility of endometriosis is almost a certainty.

- Adenomyosis, a type of endometriosis in the wall of the uterus, can be seen on ultrasound.

General Physical Examination and Non-Endo Causes of Pelvic Pain

Pelvic pain is not necessarily caused by endometriosis alone. But, pelvic pain caused by non-endometriosis conditions can exist at the same time as pelvic pain caused by endo. The following list cites causes of pelvic pain from conditions other than endometriosis and also cites common findings identified during a physical exam.

- *Interstitial cystitis:* tenderness during the abdominal exam in the midline just above the pubic bone and tenderness—or pain—when pushing on the front of the vagina and bladder during the internal exam

- *Pelvic-floor muscle spasm:* pain (sometimes severe 10-out-of-10 level) when pressure is applied with a finger on the muscles inside the pelvis

- *Psoas muscle spasm:* deep pain near the ovary and near the level of the hipbone (While pushing deep, the pain is worse when moving the patient's leg up and down.)

- *Adhesions:* pain when pressure is applied on the area of the adhesions

- *Fibroids:* enlarged irregular uterus

- *Adenomyosis:* very tender uterus that produces pain when touched

- *Uterine retroversion with collisional dyspareunia:* a tilted uterus that can be tilted back enough to become located at the end of the vagina, where it is hit during deep penetration with intercourse (The ovaries are attached to the top of the uterus and, as a result, usually drop down on top of the vagina and get hit during intercourse.)

- *Pelvic congestion:* dilation of various veins of the pelvis, especially those going to the uterus or ovaries (This causes pain around the uterus—both in general and during deep penetration with sex—and around the ovaries.)

- *Ilio-inguinal neuropathy:* painful signals from normal pressure on a nerve in the abdominal wall (This can usually be diagnosed by pushing on the tummy in the area of the nerve. The pain is worse with a crunch—tightening of abdominal muscles—done during the exam.)

- *Pudendal neuropathy:* pain transmitted to the lower pelvis including the clitoris, vagina, vulva, and rectum, through pressure on the pudendal nerve

- *Fibromyalgia:* pain on any of 18 fibromyalgia points

- *Groin hernia:* deep pain deep in the groin

- *Vulvodynia:* generalized pain in the vulvar area

- *Vestibulitis:* pain around the edge of the opening of the vagina (vestibule) resulting in pain with sex during penetration (This pain is reproduced with the light touch of a Q-tip in this area.)

- *Foreign bodies (staples, mesh):* pain in the area of the foreign body

- *Generalized visceral hypersensitivity:* tenderness, similar to a sunburn, of inside organs when touched

- *Gallbladder problems:* pain under the right rib, which is worse with a deep breath

Characteristics of a Good Endometriosis Doctor

Finding a good endometriosis doctor can be a challenge. The combination of a knowledgeable and skilled surgeon who provides care in the context of a good healing relationship is rare. Knowing what to look for is very important. The general characteristics of a good endometriosis doctor include the following:

- Knowledge and expertise in treating the various aspects of this complex disease

- Exceptional laparoscopic skills (A good measure is the percent of hysterectomies the physician does laparoscopically—as opposed to being done robotically, at laparotomy, or done vaginally. Most or all of their hysterectomies should be done laparoscopically.)

- Treats endometriosis laparoscopically with wide excisional techniques

- Listens, is non-judgmental, communicates medical knowledge in clear and understandable language, and has unwavering commitment to helping their patients

- Believes in the severity of your disease and understands that your pain is real

- Appreciates the role of a wide range of associated conditions that may be part of the pain

- Either treats a wide range of conditions (for example, pain management, interstitial cystitis, food allergies, metabolic evaluation) and/or has a network of expert health care providers that will be part of your health care team as needed

- Is open to integrative or complementary treatments

How to Find a Good Endo Doctor

There are many general OB/GYNs, and your insurance company will tell you they are all qualified to treat endometriosis. But the reality is that only a handful of doctors understand and treat this condition well. It is important to keep in mind the characteristics of a good endometriosis doctor (see the section above). Unless you have a well-known endometriosis expert locally, try to find, evaluate, and visit at least two doctors before deciding on the best doctor to help you with treating your endometriosis.

The following steps will help you find the best doctor for you:

1. Find potential endometriosis doctors.

   a. Research the web; Google potential doctors and find out everything you can. Some women will decide to travel to see a well-known endometriosis physician, while others will try to find the best local doctor to help them.

   b. Speak with endometriosis support groups to see if they have recommendations for doctors in your area.

   c. Ask nurses and operating room personnel at your local hospital or surgery center, if you have any leads or connections. They usually know who the good doctors are and who to avoid.

   d. Try to find the best laparoscopic gynecologic surgeon in your community.

   e. Get referrals from family practice doctors and gastroenterologists (bowel doctors) who you know.

   f. At the appropriate time in the process, ask to contact some of the doctor's patients who have a similar situation to yours.

2. Prepare for your first appointment.

a. Answer as many questions as you can on the "Endometriosis Physician Practice Style Assessment Form" (page 201) before making an appointment with the physician.

b. Bring any remaining questions with you to your first appointment, along with specific questions appropriate for your situation.

c. The importance of a healing relationship has been established scientifically. Gather as much needed information to complete the "Quality of Healing Relationship Assessment Form" (page 202–203).

3. Ensure a successful first visit with the doctor.

Endometriosis and pelvic pain can represent a wide range of conditions and severity to different women. Some may have moderately painful periods that are easily treated with birth control pills, while others are unable to perform basic daily tasks, with severe and complex cases causing constant excruciating pain with declining function of multiple organ systems.

a. Patients with more complex cases need to be more diligent and detailed in their evaluation process. Interview your doctor during your first visit, before he or she begins diagnosing and treating your problem. You might want to arrange this with the office ahead of time to make sure the doctor is willing to discuss the details of how he or she would interact in addressing your health care needs. It is important to make sure it is a good fit.

b. Endometriosis and pelvic pain can be complex and a time consuming process to treat. Special skills are needed to successfully treat this disease. Ask the doctor to what extent they treat endo and pelvic pain and to what extent their office is set up to deal with the various additional issues that you may need to have addressed.

c. What is their philosophy? Lupron? Laparoscopy? Coagulation? Excision? Other treatments? Make sure to also get answers to all the questions needed to complete the "Endometriosis Physician Practice Style Assessment Form."

d. How does the doctor and his office staff interact and treat their patients? Do your best to get any information you need to complete the "Quality of Healing Relationship Assessment Form."

e. Ask questions applicable to your situation, including what conditions (pain management, interstitial cystitis, food allergies, metabolic evaluation, etc) they treat in-office and if they have a network of expert health care providers that will be part of your health care team as needed (urologist, physical therapist who specializes in pelvic pain and pelvic floor muscle spasm, gastroenterologist, pain-management specialist, nutritionist or holistic health care practitioner, mind/body practitioner, sex therapist, marriage counselor, or pain psychologist).

f. Express that you appreciate and respect the time constraints of a normal office visit. How much time do they allow for an office visit? If your situation is more complex than can be dealt with in one office visit, how do they handle it? Can you book multiple visits, even in the same week?

g. Write your questions out before and bring them with you to the appointment. Take notes during the appointment.

4. After your appointment, evaluate your findings.

a. Review the entire process, including all the questions and answers.

b. Complete the "Endometriosis Physician Practice Style Assessment Form" on page 201.

c. How did each physician score (maximum is 100)?

d. Complete the "Quality of Healing Relationship Assessment Form" on page 202–203.

e. How did each physician score (maximum is 20)?

f. Did the doctor thoroughly explain your treatment options?

g. Did the doctor respect complementary therapies, such as acupuncture and meditation, rather than dismissing them out of hand?

h. Did one doctor stand out as the right one for you? Look at all of your information including the two Assessment Forms. This objective information can help you make your decision, but trust your gut feeling as well when deciding which physician is the best fit for you and your situation.

Endometriosis Physician Practice Style Assessment Form[i]

Question	Answer (Points)	Points
Does the physician specialize in treating endometriosis?	No (–10) Yes (+10)	
What percent of their practice are endometriosis patients?	0–25% (–10) 25–50% (0) 50–75% (+5) 75–100% (+20)	
Do they also deliver babies? (While a noble profession, it usually takes up too much time to specialize in endometriosis.)	No (+10) Yes (–5)	
Does the physician use wide excision (the preferred method of laparoscopic surgery) rather than coagulation? (See chapter 6, pages 90 to 116, for further discussion of surgical techniques used in the treatment of endometriosis.)	Coagulaton (–30) Limited excision (0) Wide excision (+30)	
If the physician has wide excision experience, where did the physician learn how to do to this type of surgery? (This rarely happens during training as a resident.)		0
When birth control pills do not work, does the physician routinely prescribe Lupron to treat endometriosis pain, rather than first treating it laparoscopically?	No (+5) Yes (–30)	
Does the physician work with a team? (This might include an on-site team or referrals to a urologist, a physical therapist who is specializes in pelvic pain and pelvic floor muscle spasm, a gastroenterologist, a pain-management specialist, a nutritionist or a holistic health care practitioner, a mind/body practitioner, a sex therapist, a marriage counselor, or a pain psychologist.)	No (–10) Yes (+20)	
Have women in support groups or online chat groups for endometriosis had good experiences with this doctor?	No (–5) Neutral (0) Yes (+5)	
TOTAL SCORE		

i This assessment form provides a relative scale when comparing physicians' practice style in treating endometriosis. It is not meant as an absolute scale but rather comparative only. The total possible score ranges from -100 to +100. Physicians with a practice primarily devoted to treating endometriosis providing laparoscopic wide excision will score higher on this scale, while general OB/GYNs who either primarily use GnRH agonists (for example, Lupron) or use coagulation during surgery will score lower This assessment form is intended only as a tool to help you in your search for an endo physician that is appropriate for you. This assessment tool is based on Dr. Andrew S. Cook's opinion of various factors and their importance in providing optimal care for endometriosis. It is not based on ACOG (American Congress of Gynecologists) guidelines and varies from their most recent practice bulletin.

Quality of Healing Relationship Assessment Form[ii]

Place a check in the Agree or Disagree column, based on your evaluation or experience. Each statement you agree with is given one point. Statements you disagree with are given zero points. Add up the number of points (checks in the Agree box) to get the subtotal and overall total scores. A higher score represents a higher quality of healing relationship.

Part 1: Three characteristics of a good healing relationship	Agree	Disagree
Valuing		
Physician has an emotional bond with their patients		
Physician is nonjudgmental		
Physician is fully present when interacting with the patient		
Physician is not distracted, dismissive, or critical		
Patient feels listened to		
Patient feels respected		
Patient feels valued		
Appreciating Power		
Physician consciously manages knowledge and power in ways that maximizes benefit to the patient		
Physician communicates in understandable terms, not medical jargon		
Physician clarifies procedures and treatments		
Physician encourages the patient to follow treatment recommendations for good health		
Physician works with patient as a partner in her health care		
Abiding		
Physician shows commitment to the patient		
Physician or staff returns phone calls		
Patient feels she will not be abandoned		
SUBTOTAL of Part 1 checks (total possible = 15)		

---

ii   The information used to create this assessment form is based on data in the article "Scott JG, Cohen D, di Cicco-Bloom B, Miller WL, Stange KC, Crabtree BF. Understanding healing relationships in primary care. Annals of Family Medicine. 2008;6(4):315-322"

Part 2: Patient experience as a result of a healing relationship	*Agree*	*Disagree*
Trust		
Patient is willing to be vulnerable		
Patient feels she is in a "safe" environment; she can discuss her situation openly with the physician		
Patient knows the physician will do his or her best to help her		
Hope		
Patient believes there is a better future beyond her current suffering		
Being known		
Patient feels her physician understands who she is and what she is going through		
SUBTOTAL of Part 2 Checks (total possible = 5)		
TOTAL of Part 1 and Part 2 checks (total possible = 20)		

INDEX

Entries in italic refer to figures, tables, and journals

Increase Awareness of
What it Really Means to Have Endometriosis

*Please distribute unaltered photocopies of this
two-page summary to anyone who needs an overview
of what it means to have endometriosis.*

Endometriosis is, by definition, a disease process where the inside lining of the uterus—the endometrium—flows back up inside the body around the ovaries and bowel where it implants and begins to grow. For some people, these medical descriptions can be quite dry and boring, and they do not convey what it is like for a woman to have this disease and how it truly impacts her life, her family, her career, her sex life, and her ability to live her life in very basic ways.

In reality, this disease can be like having tens or hundreds of excruciatingly painful blisters covering the inside of the pelvis. Pelvic pain and a second symptom, infertility, are the two most common symptoms of endometriosis.

Patients with endometriosis can experience horrific pain. For the lucky ones, it lasts just a couple of days during their period; in the worst cases, the pain is 24/7. The dichotomy between the way women with endometriosis look fine on the outside, but are experiencing excruciating pain internally can cause even well-meaning people to doubt the severity of their pain.

Most women begin to have pain in their teenage years, sometimes even starting in elementary school. While similar in timing, this pain is completely different from normal menstrual cramps. It is not uncommon for these girls to miss several days of school each month from cyclic pain that can exceed the level of pain patients experience after major surgery.

A lack of awareness of this disease can leave these girls without a correct diagnosis and support from their physicians. This can lead to a lack of appropriate treatment for the pain and invalidation of the patient's situation. Her family is now led to believe that psychological issues are driving the severity of her pain. In this tragic situation, she is effectively held prisoner and tortured by her own body in broad daylight, with no one who fully understands her situation or who can effectively help her.

The symptoms usually progress as she matures into a young woman. Both the severity and duration of the pain typically increase. Initially most days each month are pain-free, but the number of these pain-free days is slowly replaced by an increasing number of non-functioning pain days. The unpredictability of the increasing number of pain days makes it challenging to maintain a functional life. It becomes increasingly difficult to make plans for a future date, as it becomes more likely that it will be a pain day and she will not be able to follow through on her commitment for the activity.

As a disease, endometriosis can take away many additional aspects of a normal life. Mothers cannot reliably meet the needs of their children when the pain is too severe to function. Wives try to push through the pain to be intimate with their husbands. But eventually the pain becomes too intense to continue. Grinding fatigue, as severe as that experienced with advanced cancer, is present in most cases. Bloating, moodiness, and bladder and bowel issues are common as well.

Feeling like a vibrant desirable woman is long gone. Acting like the loving compassionate woman, mother, and partner that she truly is becomes more and more difficult. The stress on family relationships is common and real.

Even at this stage, most women fight the disease, refusing to let it completely take over their life. You would most likely pass right by them in public, having no idea of the devastation they are dealing with. Most of the time they get up, put on a brave face, and do their best to live a normal life.

The medical definition of endometriosis does not even begin to describe the reality of what it means to have endometriosis. The next time you hear about endometriosis, please remember how devastating this disease can be to a person. While endometriosis can be frustrating, if you have a loved one, friend, or co-worker who suffers from endometriosis, please remember to treat them with respect and compassion.

ABOUT THE AUTHOR

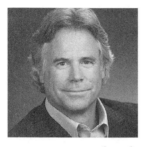

Andrew S. Cook MD, FACOG, founder and medical director of Vital Health Institute, in Los Gatos, California, is a nationally recognized women's health expert who has devoted his professional life to helping women with complex health problems. A renowned gynecologic surgeon, he is a leader in minimally invasive surgical techniques and a pioneer in the treatment and management of endometriosis.

Dr. Cook trained as both a gynecologist and a reproductive endocrinologist. He finished his fellowship at the Johns Hopkins University School of Medicine in 1991 and has been in private practice, primarily in Northern California, since then.

Dr. Cook is one of only a handful of experienced specialists devoted to the treatment of endometriosis and pelvic pain. Even among these specialists, he is unique in his comprehensive approach to his patients' overall condition.

Dr. Cook is known for his compassion, dedication, and a leading-edge integrative approach that combines traditional Western medicine and surgical treatment with complementary care and a holistic philosophy. Women from across the country and throughout the world turn to Dr. Cook for help with complex pelvic problems.

Vital Health Institute
15055 Los Gatos Blvd, Suite 250
Los Gatos, California 95032-2025
408-358-2511 or toll-free 888-256-7705
www.vitalhealth.com